TRUST *and* BETRAYAL
in the Treatment
of Child Abuse

TRUST *and* BETRAYAL
in the Treatment
of Child Abuse

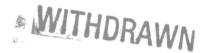

Laurie K. MacKinnon

Foreword by Virginia Goldner

THE GUILFORD PRESS
New York   London

© 1998 The Guilford Press
A Division of Guilford Publications, Inc.
72 Spring Street, New York, NY 10012
http://www.guilford.com

Printed in the United States of America

This book is printed on acid-free paper.

Last digit is print number: 9 8 7 6 5 4 3 2 1

Library of Congress Cataloging-in-Publication Data

MacKinnon, Laurie K.
  Trust and betrayal in the treatment of child abuse / Laurie K.
MacKinnon.
    p.   cm.
  Includes bibliographical references and index.
  ISBN 1-57230-298-4
  1. Abusive parents—Counseling of. 2. Psychotherapist and
patient. 3. Family psychotherapy. 4. Working class families.
5. Child welfare workers. 6. Therapeutic alliance. I. Title.
RC569.5.C55M33 1998
616.85′82230651—dc21   97-43972
                                                          CIP

Acknowledgments

M ANY people helped me develop and produce this book.

I would like to express my gratitude to all the parents and professionals who donated their time and responded with interest and openness to my inquiries into their lives. This book owes its existence to them.

In terms of the research project, I am indebted to Drs. Stuart Rees and Jan Larbalestier, both of the Department of Social Work, University of Sydney. Stuart inspired me with his unfailing commitment to qualitative research and the client's view. Jan gave me invaluable support and direction in exploring issues through sociological and feminist lenses.

Professionally, I am indebted to Kerrie James, Clinical Director of Relationships Australia, New South Wales. Our collaboration as therapists allowed the ideas emerging from the research study to be converted into concrete ideas for practice. Kerrie contributed to writing Chapters 6, 7, and 8. Her continuing encouragement and support sustained me in writing the remaining chapters.

From 1988 to 1996, the family therapy team at Dalmar Child and Family Services applied the ideas in this book to all their child-at-risk cases. Their successes with difficult cases and their unfailing enthusiasm for working by "the book" have been a source of delight and support for me. My thanks to Clive Price, David Bailey, Jacquie Tulloch, Sandra Martel, and Brett Acworth.

I would like to thank Drs. Rick Imeda and Suzanne Eggins, from the University of New South Wales, for their helpful organizational and editorial advice. Lea Chrisante, of Relationships Australia, New South Wales, read the manuscript with a critical eye for cultural and ethnic issues.

As the time line for this book extended from 2 years to several, Sharon Panulla, my editor at The Guilford Press, has been endlessly patient and supportive.

The production of this book would not have been possible at all without the exceptional skills, dedication, and generosity of June James. June took responsibility for the entire word processing of this book, transcribed all the interviews and hundreds of hours of dictation tapes, and processed endless revisions. Her interest, enthusiasm, encouragement, and constant involvement have been a great source of support to me.

The birth of my son, Sasha, midway through this project allowed me to experience firsthand the love and challenges of being a mother.

I would like to thank my mother, Frances, for her ongoing support and confidence in me. The sacrifices both my parents made allowed me the intellectual and educational opportunities I have had.

I dedicate this book to the memory of my father, Alexander, in appreciation of his nonpatriarchal style and support of my intellectual development, but mostly because I know that this work and the achievement it represents would have meant the most to him.

Foreword

LAURIE MacKinnon's deeply thoughtful and helpful book on the family treatment of children at risk is in the best tradition of family therapy. MacKinnon and her collaborators have elected to step into the space so fatefully and fruitfully inhabited by Salvador Minuchin and his team now more than 30 years ago. That classic project launched a unique tradition in our profession—a tradition of engagement with marginalized, disparaged people and with the impossible problems they present and must endure.

The impulse to take up and take on cases that professionals typically avoid or ignore is not merely humanistic, although that is rare enough. It also embodies a kind of daring and grit that has woven its way through our professional culture. Yet this taste for knowlege of (and in) "the trenches" is, once again, not simply about values and temperament. It is, ultimately, about the pragmatics of knowing. Investigators like MacKinnon are looking for an immersion experience designed to explore core questions about human relationships, psychotherapy, and social control, and to test themselves and their methods as vehicles of change and healing.

This longstanding legacy of clinical activism that combines social commitment with theoretical rigor has taken many forms as new paradigms and discourses have emerged in our field. MacKinnon's work, like many current efforts, is deeply immersed in and indebted to feminism, and to postmodern theories of knowlege and of the subject. But even as she critiques and deconstructs "the family," "child abuse," and the theories that purported to explain them, she keeps the faith by insisting that a commitment to multiplicity and uncertainty must inform, but cannot overrule, our responsibility to act both as citizens and as professionals when children are at risk of harm.

We can be glad this book pushes itself to the limits: systematically critiquing pathology-based theories of "abusive families," documenting how gender injunctions and class hierarchies create the conditions for abuse by the immiserization of family life, encouraging individual voices and stories, even when they are repugnant and implausible, yet never wavering in the moral conviction about the necessity to love and protect children, to eschew violence and domination in all its varieties, and to insist on accountability and remorse when those convenants are broken.

This generous yet uncompromising stance is arduous to maintain since the therapist is buffeted by mutually contradictory identifications and allegiances all the time. She must represent and personally identify with the family-as-victim of an overly zealous, unconsciously classist, intrusive bureaurocracy while simultanously representing and identifying with the state's commitment to overrule family sovereignty in order to protect vulnerable children from abusive parents. She must also be prepared to see and treat parents as both victims and perpetrators, and to understand and respect children's intense attachment to their parents and families, even when they are gravely hurt by them.

The therapist must be able to hold these multiple identifications in dynamic tension, even as they threaten to split the family, the treatment system, and the therapist herself. Moreover, while containing multiplicity in her thinking and affective capacity, the therapist must still be able and willing to take (and shift) positions in the real world. This means taking the heat and bearing the guilt of advocating that a father or child be removed from the home, holding a battered woman responsible for her abusive or neglectful treatment of her children, etc. In other words, she must be capable of generating and containing multiple identifications while knowing that at any particular moment, an identification with one person or position may mean the crushing abandonment of another person or another truth.

So who and what holds the therapist together as she attempts to hold onto a deep recognition of the integrity of these families, an appreciation of the contradictory facets of these embattled parents, a solemn commitment to the safety and well-being of the children, and a respectful collegiality with the other professionals and caseworkers who, like herself, are the designated advocates for society's (ever-changing) laws and values about child protection? The answer, of course, is that everyone who does this work needs brave and detailed books like this—books that in their thick description walk the walk, providing expert guidance, reassurance, and innovative technical suggestions that mobilize agency and create space for dialogue between all the parties. Especially important for the maintenance and expansion of therapeutic agency is the welcome and crucial message the book sends throughout: "This has worked for us, but may not be right for you."

Finally, we can all thank MacKinnon whether or not we have elected (or have been consigned) to do this very difficult work. Her intellectual ambition, moral perseverance, and emotional generosity shine through these pages in a way that dignifies and elevates the clinical enterprise no matter what form it takes.

VIRGINIA GOLDNER, PhD
Co-Director, Gender and Violence Project
Ackerman Institute for the Family

Contents

II. THE THERAPIST AS POWER BROKER

Introduction

THE purpose of this book is twofold. First, and most important, it represents a form of resistance to the dominant discourses that inform and construct therapists and child protection workers operating in the area of child abuse intervention. Second, this book aims to provide direction to therapists who feel overwhelmed and helpless in the face of apparently distrustful clients, and confusing and contradictory demands from child protection authorities.

The perspective from which this book grew has its origins in a qualitative research study and a therapy project. The primary aim of the research study was to identify how parents whose children were considered at risk of child abuse experienced intervention by therapists and by the frontline workers from the department concerned with child protection. Their perceptions were then contrasted with the perceptions of the professionals involved and from the accounts documented in the professional literature. I wanted to know how parents would account for their "resistance" to therapists and the conflict that emerged between themselves and professionals. The views of these people were conspicuously absent from the practice and research literature, possibly because of the tendency to see parents as "less capable, articulate and objective than other human service recipients, and ... the considerable difficulties of gaining their confidence" (Magura & Moses, 1984, p. 100).

The core of the research project centered around open-ended in-depth interviews with parents and, in some cases, children from 44 families who had experienced intervention from therapists and child protection services. Formal interviews were also conducted with 20 therapists and eight workers from the state department for child protection. The study was also informed by my involvement as a participant/observer, therapist, supervisor, and consultant to therapists working with child-at-risk cases from 1985 to 1991 in the area of Sydney, Australia (MacKinnon, 1992).[1]

Families were referred to the project primarily from public sector therapists. As is typical of child-at-risk cases referred to therapists, many of these families were socially or economically disadvantaged. Over half relied on some form of social assistance, many were single parents, and the majority, when employed, held unskilled blue-collar or clerical positions.

While I was conducting interviews for the research project, it became apparent that the information emerging from this study had important implications for the practice of family therapy. In 1987, my colleague Kerrie James and I embarked upon a 2-year therapy project in which we saw only child-at-risk cases, many of whom had been referred from or were involved with the state child protection authorities. During the therapy project, we applied the information we had gained from the research project and experimented with different approaches to the management of child-at-risk cases. Greater success in engaging parents and managing case difficulties gave us more access to the relationship context in which child abuse occurs and hence prompted us to reconceptualize the meaning and nature of abuse.

Over the last several years, the ideas that evolved from the therapy project were taken up by a team of family therapists who provided services to a predominantly lower-working-class population in the outer suburbs of Sydney. A large proportion of their referrals originated from the child protection authorities. Their success in engaging and working with families formerly considered "too hard" earned them the respect of the local department for child protection. It also demonstrated the effectiveness of this approach in the hands of both experienced family therapists and beginning family therapists working under close supervision.

This book has been organized into two parts: Part I, Child Abuse in Context, addresses how child abuse intervention is conceptualized.

Chapter 1 answers the question Why Are Child-at-Risk Cases So Difficult? by examining the larger social context of child abuse intervention and the complexities of case management that set the stage for mistrust and conflict between professionals, and between professionals and parents.

In Chapter 2, Routes to Therapy, the difficulties associated with different routes of referral to therapy are examined. Therapists encounter the most difficulty with parents whose previous negative experiences with the child protection authorities influence their subsequent willingness to trust and engage with therapists.

---

[1]For details of the methodology, see Appendix.

Chapter 3, Becoming a Client of "the Welfare," examines how families become clients of the Child Protection Department (often known to clients as "the Welfare") and how aspects of their experience with the Department influence how they are likely to perceive a subsequent relationship with therapists.

Chapter 4, Working-Class Life and the Family Ideal, counters the notion that child abuse is due primarily to the pathology of parents. Utilizing the lenses of gender and class, this chapter demonstrates how violence is intrinsically related to working-class life.

Chapter 5, The Genealogy of Relationships, looks more locally at what happens within families, how and why abuse is perpetrated, and the social discourses that underpin it.

Part II, The Therapist as Power Broker, describes an approach to working in therapy with families in which there are allegations of child abuse.

Chapter 6, Initial Meetings: Earning the Parents' Trust, outlines a number of strategies by which therapists can begin to earn parents' trust and establish a structure for later work.

Chapter 7, Working with "the Welfare," examines the relationship between therapist, family, and protective services, and how therapists can prevent problems, intervene in difficulties, and assist parents in working toward goals set by Child Protection Workers.

Chapter 8, Raising the Stakes: Eliciting and Maintaining Parents' Motivation, provides guidelines for minimizing the negative consequences of notification and for constructing therapeutic leverage in order to elicit and maintain parents' motivation throughout the course of therapy.

Using case examples, Chapter 9, Rewriting the Story of Abuse, describes the process of obtaining the story of abuse from family members and rewriting the history of their relationships in terms of the experience of power and powerlessness.

Chapter 10, Creating a Relationship Discourse, describes how therapy can elicit from family members a commitment to nonviolence, fairness, and equity and can make apologies a part of the family discourse.

In keeping with the intention of this book to give voice to the parents' experience, verbatim quotations are provided throughout many of the chapters. In Part I, quotations are drawn primarily from the research project. Names and identifying information concerning clients and professionals have been altered, and recording and transcription of their voices was done with their knowledge and consent for research and training purposes.

Case material in Part II was inspired by our experiences during the therapy project and by the experiences of therapists I have supervised over the years. To ensure privacy, however, it was necessary to construct family stories that were logically similar to but not the same as families with whom we worked. Thus, these family stories should be regarded as fictionalized accounts, and any resemblance they may have to real events or the lives of real families is coincidental. Since the therapy project reflects the joint work of Kerrie James and myself, the term "we" refers to both of us.

In keeping with my criticisms of the dominant professional dis-courses, I have tried to keep the writing accessible, the theory grounded in practice, and to avoid the mystification of "objectivity." The grounded nature of the theory also means that it is presented as local knowledge rather than grand theory. Its specific applicability to other localities and contexts will vary, but the questions it raises and the perspectives it offers should have applicability across localities.

Nevertheless, as all knowledge inevitably is, the experiences upon which this book is based are located within a particular culture, time, and place, and constructed through my eyes as a classed and gendered subject with a particular interest in and interpretation of therapy and child protection. Other therapists and researchers would, no doubt, ask different questions and construct very different answers. Even within the state in which we practice, child abuse intervention has changed considerably since the research project was completed, with a change of government, reordering of state priorities, and cuts to both family therapy services and child protection authorities. The issues addressed in this book, however, continue to be raised by therapists and reflect similar concerns to those expressed by family therapists and professionals in other states of Austra-lia, the United States, and Canada. The general themes addressed in this book are likely to continue to permeate the field in the foreseeable future in both this state and others. While specific policies concerning child protection and therapy are constantly changing and differ from state to state, the dominant discourses that underlie policy and practice are common, deeply rooted, and change more slowly.

There are many contradictions and paradoxes in undertaking therapy with child-at-risk cases, and I would not claim to have them all worked out.[2] This book provides a framework for working through some common difficulties. Each case is unique and particular, however, requiring careful thinking, planning, and review. I hope those using the ideas in this book do so with good support and review by colleagues and supervisors. This book is not, and is not intended to be, a treatise on doing therapy. The

---

[2]Other feminist family therapists have turned their attention to issues of violence in recent years and offer interesting alternative perspectives. See, for example, Goldner, Penn, Sheinberg, and Walker (1990); Sheinberg, True. and Fraenkel (1994); and Sheinberg (1992).

approach described herein presumes a certain level of skill in working with families and is written as an addition to, not a replacement for, the many skills that therapists already possess. Rather, this book was written to address a gap—a gap created by our failure to really understand the experiences of parents caught within a system they experience as oppressive and unfair. To fill this gap, we must come to terms with issues of class and gender and our privileged position in relation to the parents who are our clients.

Therapists who work with parents who have abused walk a fine line. If therapists lean too far to one side and thereby invoke judgment and social control, they risk alienating parents and losing the opportunity for therapeutic change. If therapists lean too far to the other side and do not invoke social control when necessary, therapy is potentially dangerous and risks colluding with physical and emotional damage to a child and possibly even loss of life. As Virginia Goldner has eloquently described it, working with violence requires us to maintain a position of "both–and." Violence and domination are *both* psychological *and* material, moral, and legal (Goldner et al., 1990). It is important not to minimize the effects or consequences on a child of a parent's behavior.

We, as therapists, can never be neutral either to acts of violence or to the social control exerted upon those who perpetrate harm. We are actively constructed and positioned within social and professional discourses concerning child abuse and the family. We are continually faced with choices about how to respond, and each choice carries with it a judgment about what is fair, proper, and just; the implicit taking of sides; and the use of a therapist's power and authority to alter or support current power arrangements both within the family and between family members and professionals. When our lens is focused only on what happens within the family, judgments about the fairness or justice of what happens between family members and professionals are made by default and without awareness of their implications. Knowingly or unknowingly, we are the power brokers in this drama. It is the thesis of this book that if we can more clearly understand what the social and professional discourses are and embrace, rather than deny, our position as power brokers, we can create the conditions for genuine therapy in spite of, or perhaps because of, existing within a context of social control.

PART ONE

CHILD ABUSE
IN CONTEXT

Why Are Child-at-Risk Cases So Difficult?

DURING my early years as a therapist in a family therapy clinic in Canada, I went to great lengths to avoid taking on cases involving children at risk. I avoided them not only because I found the idea of abuse repugnant, but also because the cases themselves were so messy and difficult that therapy often seemed impossible. Referrals from child protection authorities posed a series of problems for me and other therapists while consuming double the time and energy of our other work. Families were hard to engage in therapy. Arranging appointments was often difficult, as many parents earned little income and had no telephone. Families frequently failed to show up for appointments, and parents gave endless excuses as to why they could not attend. When cases did materialize, parents often said there was "no problem," volunteered little information, and seemed distrustful, angry and, resentful toward us. If therapy did proceed, we found ourselves in conflictual relationships with other professionals. Often, several agencies were involved, and each professional had a different opinion about the family and goals for treatment.

When I began to practice family therapy in Sydney (in the State of New South Wales, Australia) in 1985, I was not surprised to discover that therapists here had similar experiences. As social concern for child abuse increased, so had the number of staff employed by the Child Protection Department (CP Department),[1] and so had referrals from the CP Department to public sector therapists. As referrals increased, so did therapists' frustration. Asked to "assess" families and provide court reports, therapists

---

[1] I use the term CP Department to refer to the statutory authority mandated to intervene in situations of alleged child abuse. CP Workers refrs to the frontline workers who investigate and intervene in reports of alleged child abuse.

said they were angry at being put in "impossible situations." How, they asked, could they build a trusting relationship with parents while, at the same time, writing reports for the CP Department? Therapists argued that the job they were being asked to do should have been done by CP Workers in the first place. In response, some therapists simply refused to do assessments. Others said they would only accept cases after the Children's Court proceedings were completed.

On the other side of the fence, CP Workers appeared to be just as frustrated. Although the stated policy of the CP Department was to restore children to their families whenever possible, in reality, CP Workers had neither the skills nor the time to provide intensive casework. Yet referrals to other agencies for therapy were often unsuccessful. CP Workers with large caseloads were frustrated that therapists only wanted motivated, "middle-class" clients and would not extend themselves to child-at-risk cases. When therapists did accept referrals from the Department, however, therapists often complained that CP Workers did not accept the therapist's opinion and tried to control the case. The CP Worker's mandate to protect the child and the therapist's mandate to help the parent or family often put the two professionals at odds.

What is it about child-at-risk cases that makes them so difficult for the therapists who work with them? Within therapeutic discourse, the answer to that question is that families in which a child is abused are more dysfunctional or pathological than families presenting for more ordinary problems. The multitude of problems that arise in doing therapy are seen to be simply a result of the difficulties of effecting change in extremely dysfunctional parents. This book takes a different approach, one that argues that the issues and conflicts within these families do not represent a family structure qualitatively different from those in more ordinary cases, but, in fact, that abuse is an extension of "normal" family life.

There are other reasons why child-at-risk cases are so difficult for therapists. Many of these reasons are due to macrofactors outside of the therapist's immediate realm. While therapists cannot control or sometimes even affect these circumstances, awareness of them decreases both the therapist's perception of parents as the root of the entire problem or, alternatively, of themselves as hopelessly inadequate. Other reasons are due to minor factors—factors within the therapist's sphere of influence— and these concern the therapist's construction of the circumstances of those who abuse. Preconceptions about child abuse as pathology and dysfunction, and about the family as an idealized "unit" prevent therapists from coming to an adequate understanding of the background of those involved in child abuse.

THE SCOPE OF "CHILD ABUSE"

Child protection work is very much complicated because of the way in which "child abuse" is defined. When child abuse was first "discovered," it referred to severe physical injuries such as multiple fractures. As the conception of child abuse took hold, various other forms of physical injury and neglect were incorporated into the definition. When feminists highlighted the frequency with which children are sexually abused both within and outside the home, the official definition of abuse was broadened to include sexual abuse. Ultimately, many states acknowledged the existence of emotional abuse such as ridicule, scapegoating, and threats of loss or separation. What was once accepted as discipline, such as smacking or spanking, began to be regarded by many professionals as abuse, particularly when the parents used an implement to hit, and the incident resulted in bruising.

The definition of "child abuse" ultimately proposed by professionals casts a net broadly and, as we shall see in the following chapters, may conflict with cultural and class-based practices perceived by the individuals within it as "normal."

Defining child abuse in such broad terms has three important consequences. First, defining child abuse very broadly means that a large number of families are subjected to coercive investigations. Many of these families are then either not found to be abusive or are not found to be "abusive enough" to warrant further services (Eckenrode, Levine-Powers, Doris, Munsch, & Bolger, 1986).

Second, defining child abuse in such broad terms raises the number of mandatory notifications by professionals, and this number frequently exceeds the ability of child protection staff to investigate. As a result, the child protection system is forced to prioritize cases according to urgency. Those perceived as most urgent are investigated within days, while those considered less urgent take weeks or are never investigated. Many reports are unattended or given the most superficial screening or review (Newberger, 1983; MacKinnon, 1992).

Although legislators appear concerned enough to introduce mandatory notification, state budgets rarely reflect such a priority when funding child welfare services. Even when state budgets allow, hiring more workers does not necessarily solve the problem. Because of the stressful nature of the work and the lack of gratification inherent in it, CP Workers are frequently new graduates or inexperienced in the child welfare field. When the number of new workers in each office increases, the average length of experience in each office decreases. In the state of New South Wales, for example, when additional CP Workers were recruited in the

1980s, offices were filled with "green" workers with little professional background and less than 2 years' experience in the Department. Turnover was also high as these workers sought to leave the Department as soon as possible. From their perspective, training and support was inadequate given the overwhelming nature of the work they were asked to do (MacKinnon, 1992). As one CP Worker described it:

> "In terms of the sort of people they take in and the training that's given, it was very minimal when you consider the work that you're expected to do. Horrendous, really! The impact on people's lives for years, forever, really, with the files that are kept, the things that are written down, it has endless impact on people's lives. I found it very frightening. It's just a sense of being overworked, underappreciated, underpaid, overwhelmed by the whole context of it. The work never goes away. It's like putting your finger in the dike. That's all."

Without sufficient training and support, CP Workers are not very sophisticated in their ability to assess family situations. "Assessments" may be commonsensical descriptions of parental competence, assessed solely in terms of the mother's attributes. Often having had little training concerning cultural or class values, the CP Worker's own gender, class, and ethnicity may be taken as the norm (Aponte, 1994). When supervision does occur, it tends to be an administrative rather than a clinical task, reflecting the preoccupation with "covering your back." In the New South Wales study, CP Workers described how they avoided being accused of misconduct should a complaint arise by following procedures and guidelines to the letter of the law. Given any conflict between good clinical practice and case management guidelines, they followed procedures. As one worker put it:

> "There is also this other half of it which is 'protect your arse.' Because if you are seen not to do something, and if it could be shown that you didn't take steps to protect that kid and the kid died . . . that was always our biggest fear; supposing the kid dies and he's on our caseload. Because that happened, you know, about 6 years ago. The kid died and he had 'a thousand bloody welfarees' [sic] all involved in his life and still died because there was no coordination among the agencies, and the people didn't take seriously the mother's threats to the child."

At every level, staff feared the accusation of misconduct and the media battering that will inevitably follow the death of a child "known to the Department" (MacKinnon, 1992).

Third, defining child abuse in such broad terms prevents services from being truly therapeutic. Referring to the American context, Wolfe (1984) argues that "their only true mandate is protection of the child . . . their bureaucratic responsibilities preclude their ability, in the majority of cases, to provide some sort of systematic, targeted intervention beyond apprehension and removal" (p. 93). To deal with the overwhelming numbers, child protection work must necessarily be less concerned with family treatment or change. In New South Wales, CP Workers described themselves, in their own words, as "interventionists" who investigated, referred, and closed cases as quickly as possible. An interventionist approach, however, is constrained by the inadequacy of services to which CP Workers can refer children and families. Demand exceeds resources in many locations and it is difficult for workers to find appropriate professionals to whom to refer. These difficulties are magnified again if the case involves non-English-speaking families. As one CP Worker described it:

> "There seem to be so few resources for therapy and so many notifications that a CP Worker's response to receiving a notification is often one of 'not another bloody notification!' "

The pressure to intervene and refer, combined with the lack of available resources, sets the stage for conflict between CP Workers and other professionals.

CONFLICT AND MISTRUST BETWEEN PROFESSIONALS

The second factor that complicates child-at-risk cases is that the professionals involved tend to have conflicting agendas. Imber-Black (1988) documented the regularity with which medical, educational, and social work professionals differed with therapists and each other over how they defined problems and proposed solutions, resulting in escalating battles between families and professionals, and between the professionals themselves. In child-at-risk cases, disagreements arise between therapists and CP Workers over how to define problems and necessary changes, with the result that therapists feel frustrated, undermined, and powerless in managing cases (Berg, 1985; Viaro & Peruzzi, 1983; Spurkland & Koppang, 1985; Furniss, 1983). When child protection authorities refer families to therapists, parents often have no definite changes they were desiring other than to end the difficulties with the child protection agency, and therapists have no clear-cut criteria for treatment goals except to "transform bad parents into good parents" (Carl & Jurkovic, 1983, p. 443).

The referral of child-at-risk cases from the Department to therapists is complicated in a number of ways. The goals and process of therapy do vary from therapist to therapist. Waiting lists for therapy in low socioeconomic areas are often months long and, in the end, parents may refuse to attend in any case. In a context in which CP Workers retain both the statutory authority and the responsibility for the child's ultimate safety, relationships with therapists to whom CP Workers refer become complex and often bedeviled by conflict. The lack of clarity regarding roles and expectations of therapists and CP Workers, along with differing perspectives and conflicts of interests, creates a climate of mistrust between professionals.

Professionals often attribute the source of these difficulties to the parents. Therapists describe child-at-risk cases as "ripe for shifting alliances," with parents creating scenarios of "Let's you and him fight," or "Divide and conquer" between professionals. To circumvent such difficulties, many therapists believe that professionals involved with a case should clearly communicate and coordinate their efforts. This often proves difficult, however, as therapists working with cases describe them as open to confusion, miscommunication, and conflict (MacKinnon, 1992).

Therapists have the following long list of criticisms of CP Workers. CP Workers use extreme confrontational tactics in dealing with parents, jumping in "boots and all" and unnecessarily alienating parents in situations requiring delicacy and diplomacy. They fail to follow through with cases that warrant ongoing concern. They fail to follow up and simply let cases "fade away." They have unrealistic notions of what constitutes therapy and what therapy can accomplish. They think that therapy is a "magical solution," a way of changing people who have no interest in changing, or whose life situation is "impossible." In referring a case to therapists, CP Workers are motivated by the desire to transfer the burden of the risk to the child onto the therapist's shoulders or, alternatively, by the desire to collect evidence to use against a parent in upcoming court action.

CP Workers, on the other hand, criticize therapists for being unskilled at engaging clients and unable to achieve concrete changes. As CP Workers in New South Wales described it:

"All they [therapists] want is motivated cases, and we don't have any motivated cases and all our cases need therapy."

"The places were there, the community health centers or whatever were there, but with a lot of families that I felt needed it most, they wouldn't go. And there wasn't a lot of follow-up. If there was, it wasn't effective, and eventually you'd get this call to say the family hasn't come back, and it was your job again. I mean, what do you do?"

Many of the referrals made from the Department to therapists simply "don't take." The reasons for the difficulties in such referrals are complex and will be discussed in more detail in Chapter 3. Both CP Workers and therapists, however, appear to hold each other accountable for the loss and failure of these cases. CP Workers perceive therapists as either not trying hard enough or as insufficiently skilled to engage clients, whereas therapists perceive CP Workers as using therapy as a way of "filing down" a case and avoiding their continued responsibility in cases that warrant ongoing concern. As the following therapists described it:

> "Sometimes, I think the Department's anger with us is that we can't engage some of these people in therapy. Like them saying, 'They [therapists] are no good.' Meaning we don't keep the family in therapy or force them to come along here or whatever. . . . 'Oh, Mrs. such-and-such is not getting anything from coming along with you,' or 'doesn't want to come any more,' or 'you haven't been able to hang onto them,' or 'you haven't been helpful.' "

> "We have children referred here through the Department who are potentially physically at risk, and the Department wants us to try to do therapy with these families, quite often single mums, who really don't want to come here. And then I find out that while you're trying to work with the mum that the Department is not following up. They're not actually doing visits, and that makes me feel very frustrated . . . a feeling of having the cases dumped on us."

Conflict between the therapists and CP Workers also occurs when there is a disjunction between the legal or workplace requirement for therapists to notify and the CP Worker's decision to act on this notification and investigate. For example, therapists are often required to notify the Department of suspected cases of child abuse whether or not the child is still at risk. CP Workers, however, may not uncover sufficient evidence to warrant either an investigation or the Department's continued involvement. Therapists may believe they have made a *notification* when the Department perceives their *report* as insufficient grounds to formally act on the case. While "notifications" require CP Workers to carry out specific actions within a limited time frame, "reports" do not. As the following therapists described, the gap between these two positions poses particular difficulties:

> "The families don't want to come back here because you've sort of dobbed them in, and the Department doesn't see the situation suitable to follow up because there's not enough evidence to take it to court, and they just haven't the staff to do a lot of monitoring."

"There were numerous complaints around the clinic that home visits are not being made for weeks, you know, after the notification has occurred. That CP Workers don't go out, or CP Workers are saying, 'Oh, we can't do that, she's already in a play group. You know she doesn't require anything,' and they wind it down."

The conflict and mistrust that occur between professionals mirrors what occurs in the relationships between parents and professionals.

MISTRUST BETWEEN PARENTS AND PROFESSIONALS

The third factor that complicates child-at-risk cases concerns the mistrust that arises between parents and the professionals with whom they are involved. Parents perceive therapists as allied with CP Workers against them. This perception exists even when CP Workers and therapists describe themselves as in conflict with each other.

When arrangements for therapy are made by the CP Worker, parents usually expect (often quite accurately) that the therapist has received information about them from the Department and will hold the same perceptions, biases, and allegations. Parents also expect (often quite accurately) that therapy is not confidential. Therapists frequently share information with CP Workers, particularly if a court decision awaits the outcome of therapy. For many parents, therapy is not a safe place to acknowledge and discuss any concerns about their own or their spouse's treatment of the child. They rightly fear that openness with their concerns may leave them vulnerable to losing their children. In such a context, many parents find it difficult to begin to develop trust in the therapist. As one mother explained:

"You've got to feel you can trust people first. You've got to feel like—God! What if I say something and this person goes and tells the court? You know, this is what happens."

This sense of mistrust escalates for those parents who have previously had their children removed by the Department, for refugees who have suffered torture and trauma at the hands of government officials, and for those of a racial minority such as African Americans or Aboriginal Australians, whose community has had a long history of intrusion by a welfare system too eager to remove their children and place them into white homes (Boyd-Franklin, 1989).

Poor families who are reliant upon financial support from social services may also fear that should their situation be exposed for what it is (such as the "single" mother who unbeknownst to the officials has a live-in boyfriend), they may compromise their allotment from welfare (Boyd-Franklin, 1989).

Therapists state that their primary alliance should be with their client. When cases involve allegations of child abuse, however, workplace policies, the demands of State child protection authorities, the requirements of professional organizations, and even state laws concerning notification of suspected child abuse, confuse and complicate this responsibility. As one therapist stated:

> "With this specific family and probably with every family, I'd feel, for that moment, while I was with them, much more allied with the family. But in terms of how information is shared or how much I acknowledge a client's rights, then I'm more allied with the system."

The parents' perception of a therapist–CP Worker alliance inevitably affects a therapist's ability to work with a family. As one therapist commented, this alliance is communicated through the sharing of information:

> "These sorts of experiences can really affect your therapy, because often the parents connect yourself and the Department together. They know you share information in these cases. That can really affect how they think you're going to see them."

The sharing of information that inevitably occurs in these cases constitutes what in other circumstances would be considered a breach of therapist confidentiality. Although therapists believe that they should have verbal, if not written, consent from parents before sharing information with another agency, communication between therapists and the Department is often seen in a different light. Few therapists feel obligated to inform the family of communications with the Department, or to ask permission to give or receive information from them.

Very few families in therapy ever discover the degree to which their most intimate discussions are recorded, documented, interpreted, read, and discussed. In child-at-risk cases, however, where engagement is the most tenuous, parents are very likely to make this discovery. In court, the parents may uncover the therapist's opinion of them in the form of a court report or letter to the Department. Therapists become "information gatherers" who, in the eyes of the parents, betray them.

In cross-racial or cross-cultural situations where the therapist is of the dominant cultural background (Anglo–white), all of these difficulties are greatly compounded. First, families are likely to have a different view of what therapy means. Families who have immigrated from southeast Asian countries, for example, would have little sense of what "therapy" is about and are likely to fear the stigma of being seen as "crazy" by their relatives and friends (Lee, 1990). They are also likely to resist any attempts to view individual problems as family related and will resent a therapist who implies that a problem is caused by the family. Professional help or intervention may also be foreign to African Americans whose traditional sources of help have been other family members, close family friends, and church leaders, and who may feel attending therapy may label them as "crazy" within their community (Boyd-Franklin, 1989).

Second, the expectation of racism may leave minority cultural families less inclined to engage with the therapist. Although some cultural minorities (e.g., Hispanic) are inclined to accept the authority of the therapist despite the cultural differences, others (e.g., the African American) do not automatically accept the therapist as an authority. Rather, the therapist must earn credibility (Boyd-Franklin, 1989). This is more difficult in cross-racial situations, as many black families may react with "resistance" to what they perceive as "white institutions." This may be evidence of their "healthy cultural paranoia" developed over generations in response to racism, oppression, and discrimination (Boyd-Franklin, 1989).

For the most part, therapists do not understand their difficulties with clients as an interactional or contextual problem. The discourses in which therapists participate provide them with a less-confronting explanation.

NOTIONS OF PATHOLOGY AND DYSFUNCTION

The final factor that complicates child-at-risk cases is that professional intervention is dominated by the *disease discourse.*[2] Because professionals are immersed in the discourse that defines and constitutes their discipline, they have very little understanding of the lived experience of their clients and hold on to idealized notions of the family to which their clients compare unfavorably. In other words, there tends to be a marked gap between the discourse of the professional therapist and the everyday interpersonal discourse of his or her clients. This gap may represent the difference in knowledge and in social power, but it also inhibits understanding of the meaning that underlies family members' behavior.

The disease discourse of child abuse was pioneered by pediatric

---

[2]A discourse is a body of knowledge and the institutional and professional practices that go with that knowledge.

radiologists and other medical practitioners, and served their interests well (Wooley & Evans, 1955). As with the discovery of any new "disease," the discovery of child abuse promoted the status of its discoverers who hitherto had only marginal status within the medical hierarchy (Parton, 1985). The disease model perceives a symptom or disease as locatable within individual parents or families. At the heart of the disease model are two central notions: (1) that abuse is caused by the pathology of parents, and (2) that abuse is maintained through generations by the "cycle of abuse."

Abusive parents are viewed as inferior, inadequate, and less deserving than other parents. They are characterized as immature, dependent, self-centered, impulsive, hostile, aggressive, rigid, compulsive, and lacking in warmth, reasonableness, and pliability in thinking (Salter, Richardson, & Martin, 1985; Spinetta & Rigler, 1972; Doughtery, 1983; Tuszynsky, 1985). They are seen to be possessive and controlling, frequently displacing their anger and projecting blame onto others (Star, 1980). Such parental pathology is seen as due to the warping of parents through a failure to receive love and tolerance during their own childhood. Raising their own children in a similar manner, they perpetuate the cycle of abuse (Kempe & Kempe, 1978).

While the family systems approach is claimed to be a major advance over the individual psychopathology model, in many cases, it only shifts the level of pathology from that of the individual to that of the family. Physical abuse is seen as resulting from family systems that are disengaged, socially isolated, and lacking in loyalty, cohesion, and marital harmony (Alderette & deGraffenied, 1986; McNeil & McBride, 1979). Both sexually and physically "abusive families" are said to exhibit role reversals between parents and children, with parents looking to children to satisfy emotional needs (Martin, 1984; Cohen, 1983; Taylor, 1984). From this perspective, incest is sometimes viewed as functional, in a pathological sense, in maintaining family relationships and avoiding separation and loss (Zuelzer & Reposa, 1983; Gutheil & Avery, 1977).

Given such an unsavory definition of the parents, professionals easily attribute the difficulties that arise between themselves and the parents as simply more evidence of the parents' dysfunction. "Resistance" is seen to be evidence of primitive ego levels, rigid defense mechanisms (Salter et al., 1985), the parents' enjoyment of abusing power (Sgroi, 1982), and as being characteristic of a rigid and dysfunctional system that is unable to tolerate the threats to its equilibrium or homeostasis posed by a therapist's demands for change. These families, it is said, seldom perceive the need to change their own interactional patterns (Spurkland & Koppang, 1985) and are often willing to tolerate family breakup rather than go through the process of change in family relationships (Furniss, 1983). The notion of resistance and the lens of the disease discourse set up and maintain an interactional process between parents and professionals. When professionals maintain views of *unconscious resistance* and *homeostasis*, they adopt a posture and method that generates suspicion about what parents say, which, in turn, activates the parents' defensiveness (Ransom, 1982). By focusing on weaknesses rather than strengths and resources, professionals contribute to the parents' response and show the parents' sense of their own capabilities (Imber-Black, 1988).

When parents are referred because of child abuse, they expect that in some way they will be blamed by therapists. Their fears concerning stigma and judgment are sometimes well founded. Therapists describe themselves as wrestling with a complex set of reactions including anger and blame, and parents are finely attuned to their therapist's response. When feeling blamed, parents respond defensively by providing excuses and minimizing the effects of their behavior. Therapists may then feel provoked into taking a position seen by parents as moralistic and judgmental. As one parent, for example, described, the therapist "all but strode up and down and thumped the pulpit. . . . he made us feel like animals."

Parents often perceive therapists as blaming them whether therapists are intending to confront parents or simply attempting to understand the problem or offer alternatives to physical discipline. For parents, when the connection between the therapist's questions and the problem as viewed by the parents is not immediately apparent, parents interpret the therapist's behavior as implicitly blaming them.

Parents state that they long for but rarely experience the chance to tell "their story." They resist professionals who are seen as operating by "the book," with theories that seem ungrounded in the practicalities of life. Older women complain that young professionals lack the life experiences that would allow them to appreciate the stresses of being a mother. One woman, married for 15 years and the mother of five children, said she had little tolerance for professionals with no firsthand experiences of the stresses of marriage breakdown, financial problems, children's disobedience, and coping with a colicky infant:

> "She was very young, very young, very inexperienced, and I don't think all that university training and all the material you can read makes you the person with all the knowledge. Until you become a mother, until you become a wife, until you had to be placed in a crisis of financial strain, you have no idea what you're in store for."

Young mothers were also disparaging of professionals their own age who had spent their time pursuing education and career, as two mothers in their 20s described:

"I just treat them as if they're kids. One of the girls, she was 24. I'm not knocking her age because I'm 24 too, but she's never been married, never had kids, and I think this is about her first job, if you know what I mean. I think she has just come out of the Uni."

"She doesn't have any children, and she doesn't know anything about it. And she tells me to do things, and she hasn't even got children."

Professionals themselves are well aware of parents' criticisms, and, as one CP Worker described, realize that despite their expert knowledge, they may be perceived as lacking credibility:

"I feel a bit defensive when people say, 'You don't even have kids, what would *you* know?' You have one baby and you become an expert parent? When you have done nothing about learning of child development or family dynamics or family life cycles? You know nothing but you've got a baby, therefore you *know!* ... If you are a parent, you have automatic credibility with a lot of these people, and that is that. And if you don't have children, you don't have the credibility, and that is that."

Expert knowledge is often grounded in a theory of "the family" as a *system*, a perspective that highlights the interactional nature of problems (Alexander, 1985). When "the family" is referred to, however, as if it is an organism with biological and emotional needs, therapists make easy reference to "abusive families" and "incestuous families," and thus obscure details concerning who is assaulted and whose needs and views are dominant. A "systems" perspective may thus allow therapists to collapse the experiences of individuals and fail to note their contradictory and often conflicting interests and needs (James & MacKinnon, 1990). There is little consideration as to the effect of violence in creating particular family contexts, the effect of the therapy context on family members' behaviors, or the isomorphic relationship between "abusive families" and the gender relations prescribed by the larger culture (James & MacKinnon, 1990).

Research evidence has discredited the validity of personality typologies of parents and has provided little or no empirical evidence to substantiate the idea that abusing parents follow parenting practices significantly different from those of nonabusing parents (Gelles, 1973, 1975, 1978; Smith, 1984; Jayaratne, 1977). Nor has empirical evidence substantiated the idea that abused children necessarily go on to become abusive parents, finding that two-thirds of individuals who were physically abused do not go on to become abusive but provide their children with adequate care (Kaufman & Ziegler, 1987; Egeland, 1993; National Research Council, 1993). In fact, a greater correlation exists between child abuse and wife abuse than between abuse in one generation and in the next (Webster-Stratton, 1985). The experience of being abused as a child may be a marker for other family or environmental factors rather than a "cause" of abuse in the next generation (Milner & Chilamkurti, 1991).

Even more surprisingly, what is unacknowledged or discounted within the disease discourse is the relationship between poverty and child abuse. Economically disadvantaged families are disproportionately represented among child abuse and neglect cases known to public agencies in the United States, Britain, and Australia (Pelton, 1978; Wolock & Horowitz, 1984; Gil, 1975; Vinson, 1987). Poverty, racial segregation, unemployment, poor housing, and single-parent and stepparent households correlate with higher levels of abuse (Sack, Mason, & Higgins, 1985; Coulton, Corbin, Su, & Chow, 1995; Daly & Wilson, 1994). Abusive mothers tend to be significantly more depressed than nonabusive mothers, and their depression correlates highly with low-income and single-parent status (Webster-Stratton, 1985; Bachrach, 1983; Gelles, 1989). Material deprivation appears to transform difficulties such as alcoholism, mental illness, unemployment, and unwanted pregnancies into clear and present dangers to the well-being of children (Wolock & Horowitz, 1984; Corby, 1993; Langeland & Dijkstra, 1995).

Sociological evidence suggests that there are class differences in child-rearing practices. Parents in lower socioeconomic levels may be more punitive and restrictive, relying on authoritarian disciplinarian methods emphasizing "traditional" values rather than values that promote individuality, self-reliance, and opportunities for learning and growth (Smith, 1984; Susman, Trickett, Iannotti, Hollenbeck, & Zahn-Waxler, 1985). Family socioeconomic status also appears to be positively associated with cohesion and negatively associated with conflict (Amato, 1987). Fathers employed in professional occupations rather than service or unskilled occupations are more likely to be perceived by their children as being fair (Edgar, 1980). The link between parenting practices and social class is an important one that will be examined further in Chapter 2.

Within the disease discourse, the correlation between child maltreatment and poverty is discounted as simply a function of labeling and reporting patterns biased against the poor. It has been shown that physical injuries are more frequently diagnosed as "abuse" in poor families and as "accidents" in more affluent families (Katz, Hampton, Newberger, Bowles, & Snyder, 1986). Pelton (1978) demonstrates, however, that child abuse and neglect are related to degrees of poverty even within the same social class, with the most severe injuries occurring within the poorest of families. This raises questions about both the degree of social surveillance and the control of family relationships exerted on a relatively powerless group of people. The cycle of abuse thesis, Parton (1985) argues, is used to justify a greater emphasis on intervention into particular families. In exchange for limited material assistance, many families have their relationships scrutinized in a detailed way.

Whether poor families are more abusive or simply more subject to scrutiny, the fact remains that there are significant social-class differences between clients referred for child abuse and the professionals assigned to investigate and treat them.

The usual prescriptions for professionals working with child-at-risk cases is to simply "cooperate" with each other. Although collaboration may ease tension between professionals, it precludes the therapist from acting as an advocate for a client who appears to be unjustly treated by other professionals or the bureaucracy (see Malick & Ardi, 1981). Professionals frequently fail to realize that they are employing their socially sanctioned power within a context of conflicting interests, a context in which parents almost always have more at stake than do professionals. While professionals may feel anxious about losing their reputation or having their competence and effectiveness questioned, parents stand to lose their freedom, welfare benefits, children, and sense of autonomy as the service network becomes a further disorganizing influence on their lives (Cingolani, 1984; Aponte, 1994). Those in authority, such as therapists and CP Workers, may exert another level of abuse or oppression onto parents who are in many cases poor and ill prepared to deal with complex bureaucracies. The nature of professional intervention in child-at-risk cases can make it all too easy for professionals to replicate the patriarchal and oppressive structures in which they are attempting to intervene and change.

CONCLUSION

This chapter has examined why child-at-risk cases present such difficulties and complexities for the professionals working with them. Some of these difficulties are related to factors outside the therapist's immediate realm of control. Therapists operate within a context already constructed by how child abuse is defined and the resources allocated to deal with the problem. When professionals operate from different perspectives in what at times seems like an impossible context, conflict and mistrust between them is inevitable. Positioned between child protection authorities on the one hand and the families on the other, therapists find it difficult to define themselves in a manner that parents can trust. The disease discourse of child abuse allows therapists to blame parents for the difficulties of this work and provides little understanding of the clients' lived experience.

First, a foundation must be laid for a different understanding of the families in treatment. If we discard the notion of pathology, how are we to understand why some parents cause injuries to their children? What is the social context that produces the subjectivity and family structures that professionals have come to call "dysfunctional"? How can we begin to understand how parents, in all their diversity, experience their referral to therapy and the process of becoming a client of the CP Department? In answering these questions, we can modify our perspectives and practices in order to engage and work with these families more productively.

Routes to Therapy

ANNA Ryan was 24 when she was interviewed for the research study. She had three children, ages 8, 6, and 3. Anna was memorable because of her feisty nature and because her case highlighted the importance of understanding the route of referral to therapy. Referred to therapy from the Department after the preschool reported bruising on her 3-year-old daughter, Anna attended several appointments over the next 6 months. Although her therapist had several years of experience and was known by her colleagues for her warmth and ability to engage other clients, she could make no progress with Anna, who remained defensive and uncooperative. Anna denied that there was any problem and rejected the therapist's advice concerning behavior management of the children. The therapist felt powerless. Anna appeared to distrust and resist her completely.

This was so until, one day, two things happened. The first was an accident. After bringing Anna into the interview room, the therapist rolled up the window blinds to let in more light. When one blind became stuck, she attempted to release it. She was balanced precariously on a chair when she lost her balance and fell spread-eagled at Anna's feet. Embarrassed more than hurt, she joined Anna in laughing at her undignified folly. The second event was that the therapist told Anna that therapy did not seem to be useful and that perhaps they should finish. When she suggested terminating, however, Anna offered a problem for the first time. How could she get the children to stay in bed at night? The therapist made another appointment.

A few sessions later, Anna introduced the therapist to her "boyfriend." Although child protection authorities had considered Anna a single parent, Anna had a partner. He was the father of the youngest child, lived with the family, and was involved in care of the children. During the remaining sessions, it became apparent that Anna and her partner disagreed over management of the children and that her partner, and not Anna, had been physically disciplining the children in a heavy-handed manner. The therapist concluded that Anna had never abused her child, despite her claim to have done so when first confronted by the CP Worker.

Anna's initial presentation as a difficult and "resistant" client, and her transformation into an engaged and cooperative client, could not be explained by a change in her "personality." She had effectively had no therapy prior to this change. Nor could her transformation be explained by a change in her family relationships or life context. These had remained the same. In order to explain why Anna was "difficult" in the first place and why she became more cooperative, we had to look to her relationship with the CP Worker and the therapist, and how these relationships had been constructed by Anna's route of referral to therapy and, prior to that, to the Department.

Knowing how and why clients come to therapy reveals a great deal both about the degree of their motivation to change relationships and their willingness to engage in therapy. In the area of child abuse, the route of referral correlates with the likelihood of parents remaining engaged in therapy, the type of relationships the parents develop with child protection authorities, and the type of relationships the parents are likely to develop with the therapist. Evidence from the research study supported what we, as therapists, instinctively knew: Parents, like Anna, who are coerced into therapy make difficult clients, and therapy with them is often unsuccessful. It also, however, highlighted a perhaps more surprising fact: Therapists often have even less impact on less coerced but nevertheless "reluctant" referrals who, having more choices from the onset, consistently fail to keep appointments. Parents who are *self-referred,* on the other hand, present another set of difficulties that often bring therapy to a stalemate. This chapter examines each of these routes to therapy and demonstrates how the context of the referral from child protection authorities sets the stage for many of the difficulties therapists ultimately experience with child-at-risk cases.

Families arrive at the therapist's doorstep through either the initiative of the parents or through the initiative of another person or agency such as the CP Department. These various routes to therapy have been diagrammed in Figure 2.1.

As is evident in Figure 2.1, only for some of the self-referrals (those with only one parent, or those where both parents want to attend) and some consenting referrals (the expectant referrals) will therapy really be experienced as voluntary. So long as these clients and their therapists can come to and remain with a mutually agreeable definition of the problem, therapists generally describe being able to "do therapy" with these cases.

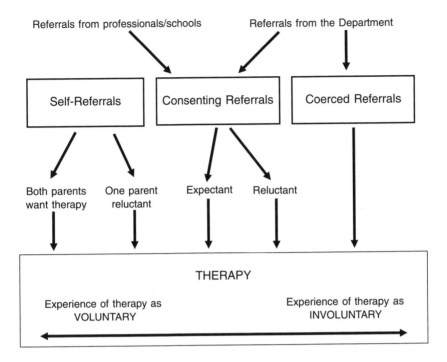

FIGURE 2.1. Routes of referral to therapy.

In the area of child abuse, however, remaining with the mutually agreed upon definition of the problem is, to say the least, often difficult, even when parents initiate therapy themselves.

SELF-REFERRALS TO THERAPY

Parents who contact therapists directly are less likely than other parents to have a history of involvement with child protection authorities or to identify their initial concern as child abuse perpetrated by a parent still living in the home. Parents will be referred to as *self-referred* when they contact the therapist directly, *without* being ordered or encouraged to do so by the Department or another professional. Some of the situations that give rise to parents contacting a therapist directly include the following:

1. Single-parent women present overwhelmed with the difficulty of raising children without adequate support.
2. Dual-parent families present with marital conflict or a child's

misbehavior. Their behavior toward the child may never have
been labeled "abusive." During the course of therapy, however,
someone discloses to the therapist that the child has been abused
or a parent's behavior becomes labeled as abusive by a parent, the
therapist, the Department, or another agency.

3. A couple who have separated seek therapy in order to reconcili-
   ate. The father may have left the home following an abusive
   incident and the mother wants his behavior or family relationships to change before he returns.

4. Parents may initiate therapy after their own child discloses being
   sexually abused by a nonresident family member or friend, or after
   a child outside the family discloses sexual abuse by the husband.

In these situations, at least one of the parents begins the relationship
with the therapist with at least some expectation that he or she can trust:
trust that the therapist will see the problem the same way; trust that
therapy is confidential; trust that therapy will help restore relationships
rather than disrupt them.

Given their initial trusting stance, it would seem that engaging
these parents should not be so difficult and, in fact, often it is not.
Problems may come later. If the therapist considers a parent's treatment
of the child to be "abusive" but the parents perceive the child's behavior
as the only problem, the therapist is propelled into a dilemma. By
focusing on family interaction without addressing the abusive practices,
the therapist risks colluding with the abuse. On the other hand, by
confronting the parents with the abusiveness of their behavior, the
therapist risks alienating the parents and losing them from therapy.
Discovering that what they considered "discipline" constitutes "abuse" in
the eyes of professionals, parents feel blamed and stigmatized, a feeling
that is compounded when parents for reasons of culture or class already
feel disempowered.

When the abuse is of such severity that it is notifiable, the therapist
faces a further dilemma. Unable to ensure the safety of children themselves, the majority of therapists agree, in principle, with the requirement
to notify. By reporting self-referred parents to the Department, however,
therapists risk losing the trust of parents who might otherwise have gained
a great deal from therapy. This dilemma is particularly acute when the
parents had asked for help from a therapist *because* they wanted to stop
abusing their child, and they are likely to feel betrayed when their request
for help initiates a coercive investigation. To make matters worse, in many
cases, CP Workers believe notifications from therapists regarding families
already engaged in therapy warrant no more than an initial investigation.
Having notified, however, therapists are left with the aftermath: parents

who no longer trust them for having made the notification and who, in many cases, subsequently terminate therapy and receive no further follow-up from either therapists or the Department.

In the area of child abuse, self-referred cases are difficult for therapists *because* they are voluntary. Their voluntary nature means that when the going gets tough in therapy, or when minor improvements are made, the parents may terminate therapy. Therapists cannot trust that the family will remain in therapy long enough to follow through with the changes that the therapist deems necessary. Therapists lack the *leverage* to ensure that the family remains in therapy and changes the behaviors and attitudes that the therapist perceives as associated with the abuse.

REFERRALS TO THERAPY
FROM THE DEPARTMENT

When families are referred directly from the Department, therapy has one great advantage: Allegations of abuse have usually been investigated and the parents' behavior clearly labeled.

Parents who are referred by the Department can be distinguished into two groups (see Figure 2.1). The first group, the *consenting referrals*, are assisted by the Department in contacting a therapist. Some of these parents have positive expectations of therapy (*expectant referrals*), whereas others feel pressured into attending and have negative expectations (*reluctant referrals*). The second group, *coerced referrals*, are ordered by the Department or the Courts to attend therapy. The parents may have no desire to see a therapist and may strongly object to doing so. Of these groups, expectant referrals are the most likely to have had a positive relationship with the CP Department and to find agreement with the CP Worker over the definition of the problem. So long as the therapist is also able to reach such agreement with the parents, therapy will seem possible. The major difficulties for therapists occur with those cases in which parents attend therapy reluctantly or feel coerced into doing so by the Department. It is useful to distinguish between these two groups, because their response to therapy is usually different.

Reluctant Referrals to Therapy

Although apparently agreeing to attend therapy, parents who are reluctant referrals may hold negative expectations of therapy and feel pressured into attending. Therapists describe them as *difficult to engage*. Shortly after commencing therapy, they sabotage the process or withdraw from contact at the earliest opportunity. Because reluctant referrals often involve a great deal of wasted time for therapists, attempts are often made to screen them out early in the process. Some therapists only accept referrals if parents telephone the center themselves and directly confirm their intention to attend. Other therapists accept referrals directly from professionals, but when parents appear reluctant to set a time or do not attend, the file is closed.

Most therapists do not regard themselves as having the time or the authority to ensure that reluctant referrals either attend therapy or stop abusing their children. When referring CP Workers are informed that the parents terminated prematurely, however, it becomes apparent that the CP Worker has gone on to other more urgent cases or can offer no further action, as these therapists described:

> "Subsequently, I had no contact with the CP Worker despite numerous attempts of mine to find out what was happening with the cases. . . . The CP Worker never got back to me, and the family dropped out and the case faded away."

> "The parents might come for a couple of times, then drop out, and we don't have any power. Get back to the Department and then they sort of say, 'There's not much we can do,' and yet I still feel the children are still potentially at risk."

Although reluctant referrals are pressured into therapy by a concerned CP Worker, they often face no real consequences such as removal of their children if they do not attend. CP Workers may claim, for example, that they can threaten no further action either because the situation is not considered serious enough to threaten removal or because the child in question has already been removed. In this way, reluctant referrals very often slip through the cracks and ultimately receive very little in the way of help from either the Department or therapists. Therapists never get a chance to show these parents that they are worthy of their trust, and they have little leverage to motivate parents to attend sessions.

Coerced Referrals to Therapy

Whereas reluctant referrals simply drop out of therapy, coerced referrals are more likely to continue to attend. Faced with serious consequences such as loss of their children or criminal charges if they fail to comply with an order for therapy, these parents, like Anna Ryan, feel they have no real choice but to attend. Nevertheless, they are often unwilling to discuss their situations openly. Although the coercion they experience ensures their physical presence in the room, it also overshadows any potential motivation to address individual or family issues, as these parents revealed:

"The judge said that I had to return to court myself on July 30th, which I did, and I was allowed to have my son back if, this is where it stinks, if I would have counseling for 2 years through some little upstart named Teresa. She's 26. I don't know what she's done in the way of training. She's not at all sympathetic, or empathic, or whatever the word is."

"How did I end up coming here? This is what I have to prove, see? They're making me. I've got a choice. Either come here and see Ken and do all these sorts of things or they take the kids away. That's the choice!"

"He just said he would see us again and we would have to come [to therapy], otherwise 'there are ways of making you come' if you don't want to come!"

Parents who are coerced referrals to therapy perceive therapy to be an extension of the CP Department and therapists, therefore, as untrustworthy. They expect that the therapist is allied with the CP Worker against them, an expectation that exists even when CP Workers and therapists describe themselves as in conflict with each other. Issues concerning confidentiality of information and the possibility of renotification often loom large for both therapists and parents.

Therapists describe coerced referrals as unmotivated and resistant, and may conclude that by ordering the family to therapy, the CP Department is shifting the burden of responsibility for the child's safety to the therapist. Therapists know all too well that therapy is not a magical solution, particularly for those clients who have no interest or desire to be there. As one therapist described it:

"I'm afraid that we take on a family into therapy prematurely and the court doesn't have full information. All the information they have is that the family is in therapy, and they write it off. I think there is a general feeling that therapy is magic and fixes everything up. It's just the buck-passing process that concerns me. In some cases it can be a very risky situation."

It is difficult and stressful, on the one hand, to have unmotivated clients, and on the other, to feel significant responsibility to "come up with the goods." Therapists want clients who "want to be there" and who show some interest or desire to talk about their difficulties. This expectation, however, feeds into the evolving difficulties between therapists and parents, as one mother described:

> "They [therapists] expect things of you; they shouldn't expect things of you. For a start, they shouldn't expect you to be happy or anything like that when obviously the situation—they expect you to be cooperative . . . they expect you to be willing to be there when they know darned well you're not . . . before you even walk in there, before they've even seen you, they must know you're not going to be quite as cooperative, you know? Well, there you go, why do they expect you to be cooperative and willing?"

In the case of coerced referrals, there is sufficient leverage to ensure the parents' physical presence in the room. But the transition from physical presence to open and active involvement in the process of therapy is difficult and often just does not happen. Parents remain in a defensive position and see little to gain in changing their behavior. Without a sense of choice, without the ability to define the problem in their own terms or have their definition of their relationship between themselves and the Department stick, these parents do the only thing left to do while preserving a sense of their own integrity: They resist. This resistance is sometimes subtle and sometimes overt, but always it is with such tenacity that child abuse cases are infamous among therapists for their difficulty.

And so we are left with the question "Why?" Why do parents find the situation so threatening that they resist us with such tenacity despite our genuine and often altruistic desire to help them? Why do they resist us so much more than other clients? The answers to these question are complex and multilayered, but in the next chapter, we will deal with the reason the parents themselves most often give: They see therapists as aligned with CP Workers and they feel blamed, stigmatized, and oppressed by their experiences of Department intervention. When parents have been referred from the Department to therapy, the background context that informs the parents' relationship with the therapist is their prior and ongoing relationship with the Department. This was the case with Anna Ryan, whose story of coercion into therapy began this chapter.

〰

CHAPTER THREE

Becoming a Client
of "the Welfare"

ANNA Ryan's relationship with the CP Department (known by many clients as "the Welfare") dated back 6 years to a time when she, at 18, was left on her own with a baby and toddler following the death of the children's father in an industrial accident. With no support from her family or his, she desperately needed a break from the children. She asked for help from the Department. When none was forthcoming, Anna believed she was perceived by them as a teenager "only wanting a good time". Some months later, Anna suffered a "nervous breakdown" and was hospitalized for a few months. Her children were taken and put into temporary foster care. Anna agreed to this placement and voluntarily signed a form agreeing to a 3-month placement. When she recovered and left the hospital, however, it took her 14 months to convince the Department to allow her children to come home. She believes that the CP Workers looked down upon her because she was young, she lacked education, she was dependent on welfare, and "They think two parents are better than one."

When, 5 years later, Anna encountered a CP Worker at her door, she envisioned losing her children again. She felt enraged at what had happened to her before, at whoever (and she suspected the preschool) had notified the Department this time and not even spoken to her, and at the CP Worker who now threatened to remove her children unless she cooperated.

Confronted by the CP Worker about the bruising, Anna retorted, "Yes, I hit her, I belted her . . . so what are you going to do about it!" The CP Worker experienced Anna as angry and intimidating, and Anna's behavior toward the CP Worker confirmed the CP Worker's perception of Anna as someone capable of child abuse. After several angry encounters with Anna, the CP Worker took the matter to the Children's Court. Despite Anna's refusal to acknowledge any problem, she was ordered to attend counseling. Anna knew that this therapist communicated openly with the CP Worker. Although she did not understand what was to happen with the Children's Court, she knew that proceedings were not finished and that both therapist and the CP Worker were likely to be reporting back to the court.

Hearing Anna's story of her experience with the Department and how she was referred to therapy makes sense of Anna's "resistance" to the therapist and to her change of position when offered a genuine choice to not attend therapy.

Parents who are referred to therapy from the CP Department may, like Anna, have had a long and complicated relationship with the Department or only a recent and short-lived encounter. For parents who are referred from the Department to therapists, three aspects of their experience with the Department influence how they are likely to perceive a subsequent relationship with a therapist: (1) the parents' route of referral to the Department, (2) the experience of being notified and investigated, and (3) the experience of court proceedings. These factors are not, in fact, separate and distinct, in that involuntary clients are more likely both to have been notified and to have been involved with the Courts. Given the impact of these experiences, however, it will be useful to consider each separately.

ROUTES OF REFERRAL TO THE DEPARTMENT

Not all parents who become clients of the Department perceive their involvement as involuntary (see Figure 3.1). Two of these routes are experienced as more or less voluntary: the *self-referrals* and the *consenting referrals*. Self-referrals contact the Department directly by either telephoning or presenting themselves at a Departmental office. When they are identifying themselves (e.g., rather than a partner or a neighbor) as the abuser, women are much more likely than men to ask for help. Consenting referrals, on the other hand, make contact with the Department as a result of a referral from another professional. Like those referred to therapy, consenting referrals can be either expectant or reluctant. Figure 3.1 diagrams these various routes to the Department. *Expectant referrals* have high expectations of the help they will receive from the Department, whereas *reluctant referrals* are more likely to have consented to a referral in order to appease an apparently helpful professional or other person. It is important to remember that parents with a longer or intermittent relationship with the Department, such as Anna Ryan, may have experienced themselves at different times as being both voluntary and involuntary clients.

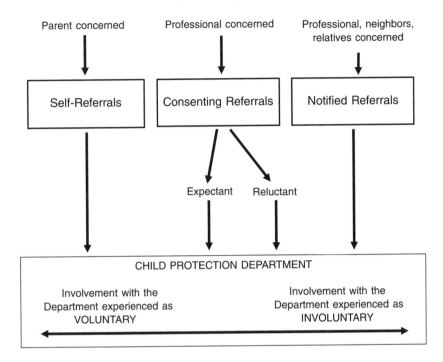

FIGURE 3.1. Routes of referral to the Department.

Voluntary Clients of the Department

Women are more likely than men to seek help from the Department, more willing to identify themselves as abusive, and more likely to remain clients of the Department. In part, this is because women remain the central cog upon which the responsibility for the care of children and relationships falls. Women are constantly comparing and evaluating themselves in this area, and the experience of failing is acutely felt. Women remain more aware of, and take more responsibility for, children and the relationship between children and their fathers than men do for children or for the relationship between children and their mothers. As documented in the following chapter, women have much to fear in terms of male violence directed toward them and their children, and they generally lack both the physical prowess and psychological makeup to ensure their safety by threatening violence in return. Women need support and allies, and they turn to the Department to obtain both.

In situations where parents initiate contact with the Department or consent to the referral, the relationship that develops with the child protection authorities is less adversarial. These parents are much more likely than involuntary clients to perceive their CP Workers as "friends." "Friends" develop "real relationships" with parents, conveying respect and advocating on their behalf to obtain needed resources. Parents experience themselves as more than just "clients" and believe they hold some personal meaning to the CP Worker, as these two parents described:

> "He tells me to get off me butt and start bloomin', to get out and do something, you know? . . . He'll sit down and have a cup of coffee with yer, he'll talk, he'll joke, but even though he's jokin' with yer, and he's friends with yer. . . . "

> "You still know not to cross 'im. You know there's a relationship there, put it that way. Yeah, there is a relationship there between us."

The subtleties of such relationships mean that they are far less likely to develop when language or cultural barriers exist as, for example, when the therapist is of a different racial background than that of the client.

Friends seem "human," willing to reveal some of their own personal experiences, including difficulties they had in raising their own children. They seem warm and trustworthy, as Myra, 24, described, referring to an incident that happened when she was hospitalized for depression:

> "That's where I first met her, in the hospital. And she was talking to me. And I started crying in hospital, and Joan came up and put her arms around me and said, 'You know, you're my first big case. You can't mess it up, you can't do this!' And she laughed and, you know, she was really human. She wasn't someone who stood back and looked and said, 'I'm Welfare and . . . now you'll do as I say or I'll take your kids.' She was actually wanting me and the kids to get together. They're human. Joan admitted to me . . . she's made mistakes, you know? Whereas Welfare people *never* make mistakes."

Voluntary clients have one great advantage. They have more influence over when and where their first meeting with a CP Worker is to occur. If they choose to go to a Departmental office to discuss their concerns, they have the advantage of more easily controlling what aspects of themselves to reveal to a CP Worker than if the Worker arrives unexpectedly on their doorstep. Despite this advantage, the experience in a Departmental office can be intimidating, an experience that elicits a sense of social inferiority, a sense of being a "lower person," as one mother described:

> "I don't want to go there by myself because I know what it's like. You just go the Department. They treat you like . . . they just leave you

in the office for ages. You sit there and waiting for them to do what they think is right. Just how they treat you. Just like a bit of dirt. I just don't like it. It's because of the way they speak to you, as if you're a lower person anyway. When you start to fire questions at them and want to know why things are happening, they sort of cut you off altogether."

If they choose to telephone to initiate contact with the Department, they are likely to wait days or weeks for a CP Worker to visit their home. When contact with the Department is made in order to protect the children from someone outside the home, waiting for the CP Worker can be experienced as unbearable. Having reported the abuser (e.g., an ex-husband, family friend, or neighbor), the parent and child may live in fear of the abuser's retaliation, as this mother described, referring to her ex-husband's potential for violence after she reported his physical abuse of their eldest son:

"It was difficult waiting, because we didn't know whether they'd been to see him or not and it was, 'Oh, God, if they'd been today, we were bound to get it tonight. . . . ' "

When, 9 days later, she had not heard from the Department, she telephoned and was told:

"They would come around. . . . They didn't come the day they said they were going to come. They came either the next day or the day after, and we didn't know whether they'd been to see him or whether they would come to see us first. . . . Anyway it was pretty scary."

Whether waiting in an unfamiliar office or enduring a seemingly unending wait for the CP Worker's arrival, parents are often intimidated and confused. They may have little understanding of welfare services, no concept, as one father stated, of "divisions within divisions," a confusion compounded when the parents are of a minority language or culture. Many are uncertain and confused about the roles of different professionals, sometimes perceiving the Department and therapists as part of the same organization, as did these mothers:

"I wasn't sure who Mr. Laren was with. I knew he worked for the Government, but I don't know if it's part of the CP Department or, even now, because I've never thought to ask the question. I don't know if he's part of the CP Department or if they're a branch of their own. . . . I see them combined."

"She was doing something with—she wasn't actually a strict member, a staff member—she was doing something, she's not with Family Home Support, and she wasn't actually with the CP Department. . . . I never ever found out what her full title really was. She had a card and everything."

When initiating contact or accepting a referral to the Department, parents have in mind a certain kind of help or solution to their problem. They are proposing a certain definition of a problem situation and asking for a response that will fit within that definition. Some parents believe they require instrumental or tangible solutions to their difficulties: child care, temporary foster care, or a move within public housing, for example. Even when the investigating CP Worker perceives the solution similarly, and frequently they do not, these parents are competing for resources in a context of high demand and few resources. Expecting service from the Department, they are disappointed and often angry when the Department either does not have the resources or determines that they are not deserving of the resources that do exist.

In a context of inadequate resources, even those parents who are seeking only to change their own abusive behavior, may find that *because they are asking for help*, they are *perceived to be* less risk to their children than those involuntary clients who are notified. Such was the case with Anna Ryan when she first asked for help at age 18, and also the case with Julie Black, 32, the mother of five young children under 12. Julie described how, when she had been investigated by the Department on previous occasions, she had feared losing her children and had explained away their bruises and fractures as "accidents." When her eldest son was diagnosed with a life-threatening disease, however, Julie became determined to stop abusing her children:

"I thought, 'This just can't continue for years, it's just not the answer. You've got to do something about it. Somebody's got to do something about it,' and so I thought I would take the first step."

When she approached the Departmental office in her area, however, the CP Worker appeared to dismiss her concerns and the severity of the situation. Although she tried to convince him that her children were genuinely at risk, she believes her situation did not receive the attention and follow-up that was needed:

"I said, 'Look, if you don't do something, if you don't take them away or do something for a while, I'm going to end up killing one of them.' And they said, 'Why, are things really bad?' And I said, 'Yes, we can't live in one house.' . . . It was really bad. It would be nothing for me to drop John on the floor and kick him. . . . I threw John against a brick wall and broke his arm. Welfare didn't do a bit. They didn't believe me. They were stupid. . . . Nobody knocked on my door and asked me what happened . . . I've been in this town for 12 months and child welfare hasn't bothered to be at my house once to see the children. They've had reports about me bashing those children. Why haven't they got off their backsides and come and seen the children? . . . I definitely wouldn't go back there again, no way!"

The nature of child protection work (the emphasis on crisis, reliance on surprise visits, and the prioritization of cases) works against many voluntary parents. Women who admit abusing their children and initiate contact with the Department may be taken less seriously and given less attention than involuntary clients who maintain they need no help. This does not mean, however, that they are, in fact, less abusive, as Julie Black's story grimly conveys.

Voluntary clients who believe they have been assisted by the Department will respond optimistically to a referral for therapy. Those who have been disappointed, however, may fear that a referral to therapy is simply further evidence of "buck-passing." They may fear being treated again like a "lower sort of person" and worry that their very-often real material needs have been reduced to psychology.[1] If, however, they encounter therapists who are empathic to their experience with the Department, who treat them with respect "as an equal," who take seriously their material concerns, and who stick with them, they will become willing and involved clients.

Involuntary Clients of the Department

Parents become *involuntary clients* of the Department in one of two ways. First, they may reluctantly accept a referral from a professional to the Department and discover, once the notification has been made, that they cannot easily retreat from the Department's involvement. The professional making the referral may have portrayed the Department in positive terms in order to gain the parents' compliance. Once in contact with the Department, however, the parents may experience the Department as

---

[1]Workers with racist attitudes may view the parents' "ethnicity" to be the cause of the problem when the parents are struggling with poverty, as was the case in Australia of the generation of lost Aboriginal children who were removed from their parents during the 1960s and 1970s to "better" white families.

coercive and bureaucratic rather than caring and helpful, as this father, whose daughter was sexually assaulted by a close family friend, described:

"It was like a military action. Like—'We're coming, we want to set a time—you be there with the child.' I was saying, 'Hang on, this is our child you're talking about! Who are you? We'll accept your help but we'll make the decision.' I really went off my head. . . . We feared the end result of this mechanized thing churning away. The way people shoved things in and out of trays, stamping and saying, 'Right, we'll go and see them.' We still felt very much like we'd gone from being complete parents to pieces on a chess board and to being pushed whichever way suited the occasion. . . . Already this sort of machine had started churning, and we felt we were under pressure. And the whole thing was going to be taken out of our hands, and we had no say in it whatsoever."

The sense of "no say in it" is shared by *notified referrals* to the Department. These are parents who, in their own words, are "dobbed in"[2]; that is, they are notified by someone outside of the family and investigated by the Department as a result of the report. The notification may have been made by a teacher, doctor, other professional, neighbor, or relative who suspects that a child has been mistreated. Notified referrals are constituted within a relationship to CP authorities, that is, from its onset, adversarial.

With both *notified* and *reluctant referrals*, the parents' first contact with the Department frequently occurs on their own doorstep. Since this "meeting" usually occurs without advance warning and, in the case of notified referrals, without consent, parents have less choice about what aspects of their lives they are to reveal. From the Department's point of view, the lack of warning is important. CP Workers are seeking to assess families in the most "natural" of situations, as one CP Worker described:

"Part of that is motivated by you needing evidence to go to court, and you only get evidence when you catch people in a crisis, and they're not going to sit there and say, 'Yeah, I beat him up.' Some of them do, but very often you get people who are so terrified they never tell you anything. So you have to catch them in the act of doing what you suspected they have been doing all along and then have a conversation with them that you put into evidence, that you then present to the court."

---

[2]Getting "dobbed in" is Australian slang for being informed on for alleged offenses to an authority by one's peers. It connotes a vindictive or retaliatory act.

Because home visits are more likely to occur during the day, CP Workers are more likely to encounter women than men. This fact is very well known to CP Workers who are less threatened by a potential encounter with a woman than by her potentially violent husband. In the case of a racial or ethnic minority family, men may be at home during the day given their unemployment, and extended family members such as grandparents and adult siblings may also be present.

For parents of either gender, being assessed within their home feels like an invasion and violation of their privacy. They do not understand clearly the role of CP Workers, what they want, or what the consequences could be of refusing to cooperate. Men and women often respond differently, however, to this threat. Men may order the CP Workers out or even threaten them physically. Women are more likely to feel powerless, intimidated, and confused, and to comply with the investigation out of fear and deference to authority. As these mothers described it:

"I didn't quite know who she was or where she was from, or what. . . . Oh, I felt terrible. I felt really . . . not abused, but my security infringed upon. They'd sort of taken away that. It was a real intimidation that I felt that—how dare they! That they intrude on our privacy, and I know when logic told me that's what they have to do, but the experience was . . . I was really taken aback."

"They came up to my house. I didn't even know why they were coming or anything, and they had this form already made out so that if I didn't hand the kids over to them, you know, I would be up for jail or a fine or something like that. . . . They didn't even give me a chance to explain."

Although allegations of abuse sting parents of either gender, it stings them differently. Men who are "heavy-handed" with children are not likely to experience themselves as less masculine for doing so. Even allegations of sexual assault are unlikely to challenge a man's sense of his masculinity. For men, the challenge from the Department is more likely to be experienced as an external threat, either trivial, as something to be dismissed or, when involving legal consequences, something to be fought aggressively.

For women, however, getting "dobbed in" is an explicit criticism of their ability to mother, and this criticism of an ability that is supposed to come "naturally" negatively connotes them as women. Women thus feel more stigmatized by being perceived as a client of the Department. They feel judged as inadequate, out of control, and unable to manage: to have failed as a mother. This sense of stigma is enhanced if the case is formally registered and continues, even if help is eventually forthcoming from the Department:

> "I suppose it's just the old reputation or stigma that's still around, or that I still felt, anyway, . . . just being out of control, not being able to look after your family and having to have someone else come in and do it for you. Afterwards, it was a bit of relief, finding that someone was doing something, and that people realized I needed a bit of help. At the same time, I felt really guilty that I couldn't do it myself."

> "Apparently, when you're on a child abuse register, you're on that for 12 months and very closely watched by the Department is what I've since been told. I was taken off that list—that *bad* list *(laughs)* last December, and I can't tell you what a relief it was. Oh, it was such a relief! Just like a whole burden had been lifted off me!"

The "bad mother" message may also be conveyed by CP Workers directly, as in the following two examples. In the first, Janet Simpson felt blamed by the CP Worker for failing to protect her 15-year-old son from sexual abuse by a neighboring adolescent boy.

> "They sized us up as uncaring parents—'but look, this has been going on for 2 years and you've done nothing about it.' . . . She constantly kept ringing me up and saying, 'What kind of mother are you?' And suggesting things I ought to do because I was an 'uncaring parent.' . . . And, ah, she reminded me before she went that I was not a good mother. And I objected to it very strongly, because if I'd known I would have acted, but when you don't know, what can you do?"

In the second example, Susan Sinclair, 24, had been notified to the Department after she had expressed to her baby health nurse her fantasies of throwing her 2-month-old twins out the window. She recalled that the CP Worker, a young woman with no children of her own, was enthralled with the twins and did not take seriously Susan's stated need for a break. Instead, she determined that there was "something wrong" with Susan, because she was not "enjoying being a mother."

> "She was on about 'I should really enjoy being a mother,' just enjoy that. I felt that she couldn't see my point of view. . . . I reckon they should have really tried hard to get some child care for me. I don't think I needed to see a psychiatrist. I think that just talking to someone, like just talking to someone would have been pretty good. But I needed some action, I needed something to happen, and it didn't."

Although the CP Worker visited Susan twice in the ensuing week, no child care was ever organized. Instead, Susan was referred to a psychiatrist who prescribed antidepressants when, as Susan said, "I knew all I wanted was a bit of child care. A bit of a break and I would have been a lot better."

For women to accept the Department's intervention is to accept that they have failed, either failed directly as mothers or indirectly, in their ability to attract and keep satisfied a reliable man and thus create an ideal family. Women who already perceive themselves as having failed in these areas by virtue of failed marriages may feel they have little left to defend. When, in the midst of an acute life stress such as a recent separation from a long-term, violent marriage, women are often more hopeful of receiving help and tend to respond cooperatively to CP Workers.

Women who have only recently experienced independence from their families of origin, however, and are perhaps still jaded by the authority structure there, are less likely to so easily accept a negative connotation of themselves, or to relinquish their newfound autonomy to be controlled or told how to live their lives. Older women still in marriages are also less likely to easily accept this negative evaluation of themselves, their husbands, or their families. Like the younger, rebellious mothers, the Department's interventions contravene their notions of family privacy and their right to discipline children as they see fit. Unlike younger women, however, they often have age, greater resources, and assertive husbands on side.

In addition to the greater sense of stigma, invasion, and loss of control, involuntary clients of the Department are likely to have three experiences that will profoundly alter their attitude and affect their attitude to therapists and professionals in general: (1) the impact of notification, (2) the process of investigation, and (3) the experience of court proceedings.

THE IMPACT OF NOTIFICATION

Parents who are "dobbed in" are left to deal with the impact of the notification on their lives. First, they must come to terms with the fact that someone they know has reported them. They often suspect or believe they know who did so. Although CP Workers are required to ensure the confidentiality of the person who notifies, details are often revealed—an inexperienced worker inadvertently discloses the identity of the notifier, a parent confronts a suspected notifier, or the case reaches court, where the names are not withheld. Even when parents are never told who notified, they often believe, rightly or wrongly, that they know. There are a limited number of people in contact with the child, and parents often deduce who would have the motivation to notify.

The closer or more personal the relationship between the parents and the assumed notifier, the more the parents feel betrayed. A notification is a declaration of someone's judgment not only of the parents as unfit, but also of the fact that the parent is not the sort of person who can be approached directly and helped or reasoned with. The sting of the notification is thus felt less intensely when acquaintances or distant neighbors notify than when the assumed notifier is the parent's ex-husband, sister, or parent.

When a professional has notified, the extent to which parents feel betrayed is related to how close or personal the existing relationship was prior to the notification. Parents who take their baby to the emergency department of a hospital, for example, harbor little resentment toward hospital personnel who notify. Parents who go to a therapist, on the other hand, asking for help in dealing with a child's misbehavior, feel angry and betrayed when the therapist notifies the Department and are likely to respond by dropping out of therapy.

Notification by day-care centers or schools may also result in the same sense of betrayal. When a child remains at a center or school following a notification, the relationship between the parents and the school or center becomes strained. Mothers feel distrusted and criticized. Parents do not believe that school officials should involve themselves in family matters. As Anna Ryan described, referring to the preschool notifying the Department because of a bruise on her daughter:

> "The preschool teacher ... didn't ask *me* about it—didn't ask *me* where it was from, and went round and told them, 'She must have done it,' or 'If she didn't she is a slack mother and just doesn't know and she ought to watch them better,' or something like that. Anyway, who cares? It was my fault that the 'proof' was there and that's what's happening now."

The feeling of being judged and the erosion of trust is not confined to the relationship between the parents and assumed notifiers but may extend to the school and extended family relationships. In order to talk to a child apart from the family, the CP Worker may arrange for an interview with the child to be held at the school. Teachers are thus made aware of the investigation. Due to "confidentiality," however, they may not be informed of the allegations or the outcome of the Department's investigation. They may not even know, for example, that the perpetrator was someone outside the family, or that abuse was not substantiated, leaving them to suspect the worst.

When extended family members become aware of a notification, they may behave in ways that parents experience as judgmental and ostracizing. This often occurs at the very time that parents need the most support. In Flo Park's case, for example, a neighbor had observed an incident in which Flo had yelled at her two children and hit one of them. He contacted Flo's ex-husband, who called the Department. Flo and her children were interviewed by a CP Worker, who determined that the children were not at risk. When Flo's sisters, however, heard of the notification through the ex-husband, they became distrustful and critical of her. Flo's already tenuous connection to her extended family was unbalanced, leaving her more isolated. Flo lamented that, because of the notification, her sisters turned against her and sided with her ex-husband:

> "I've still no maintenance. It's nearly 4 years, no maintenance, nothing. He doesn't see them, and I am hurt, I am very hurt that my family was so weak and so gutless that at the slightest thing they turned on me. And it hurts, it still hurts."

The notification may escalate extended-family conflicts, confirming a negative evaluation of a parent or the parents' relationships. The "hurt" of compounded betrayals takes its toll. Parents become defensive, angry, and less able to trust again. This accounts for some of their "resistance" when they ultimately encounter a therapist.

The second way in which a notification affects the lives of parents is related to the fact that a notification initiates the creation of a file. Files record notifications (i.e., allegations of abuse) whether or not these are ever found to be substantiated. An assumption of guilt underlies the existence of a file. A history of notifications, itself, is often taken as evidence of the parents' failure, as is apparent when one professional comments to another, "The Department has a file on them *this* thick."

The existence of a file is a black mark against the parents in the eyes of both Departmental workers and any agencies who know of the file. Parents who are "known to the Department" through previous notifications experience the Department as "big brother," who maintains an ever suspicious, "watchful eye" over them. Anna Ryan, for example, maintained that the reason the bruise on her child's leg was interpreted as evidence of abuse was because the preschool knew that her children had previously been fostered and that she was "on file." She could only conclude: "Even if this blows over, they'll keep me on their file and keep a watchful eye."

The Department sought to remove Lynn Pitman's daughter after Lynn's male partner had struck her. In arguing to the Courts for removal, the CP Worker concluded in her report that "there have already been three notifications" concerning the daughter. The report failed to mention that two of these notifications had been made by Lynn herself, a few years earlier, when she feared that her ex-husband might be sexually assaulting her daughter.

The sense of being judged and the resistance to being controlled arises again during the process of investigation.

THE PROCESS OF INVESTIGATION

The process of investigating child abuse allegations sets the stage for the difficulties later faced by therapists attempting to engage parents referred from the Department. It is during the investigation that parents first begin to resist. They do so, first, because the relationship that develops between them and the CP Worker is one in which they feel judged and blamed. Second, they perceive CP Workers as siding with children against them. Third, they feel caught in a "catch-22" about admitting responsibility for the abuse.

The process of child abuse investigations constructs for both parents and CP Workers a context that is, in most cases, adversarial. CP Workers are obligated to protect the children, even if this means removing them from the family. Parents stand to lose their children, control over their lives, and perhaps they may even face incarceration.[3] CP Workers know that parents are likely to minimize, if not conceal, aspects of themselves and their situation. In asserting their authority, CP Workers hope to achieve the parents' compliance. Parents, however, feel judged and blamed. CP Workers may be experienced as aggressive and unfriendly, providing little information about what they are doing or why. One father likened them to the Gestapo:

> "This woman—the Gestapo lady, we call her. . . . The CP Department, all they do is hinder your recovery. They don't know what they're talking about. They don't know how to do things, and the people they send out have no training whatsoever."

When lacking in-depth knowledge of the parents' circumstances, CP Workers can only make assumptions based on the parents' behavior, material circumstances such as housekeeping, and the degree to which the family appears to differ from the ideal family. Parents say they feel

---

[3]Imagine the experience of torture or trauma survivors or refugees who have already experienced incarceration, and who have gone to great lengths and expense to reunite their families over a long period of time.

categorized and judged according to normative standards. Single women may feel this acutely, as the following mothers described:

> "Because they just treat you in a certain way, like they'll say, 'Most people do this and most people do that,' and all this sort of thing, like as if I'm 'most people.' They've got a basic way of how people act and live, and they just think that everyone's like that."

> "He didn't give a damn about how the kids felt or how I felt; he didn't care. That's what I mean by the 'book.' Kids should have two parents and all that sort of thing. At the time I was living with my husband now, but we weren't married. He didn't seem to go much on that, plus he wasn't the kids' father, you see?"

> "And they asked me who I slept with, and I don't think it's got anything to do with Jenny. They haven't got the right to go asking that sort of thing. But there's nothing I can do about it."

"Assessments" often boil down to culturally embedded descriptions of the mother's character and motivations (MacKinnon, 1992; Vinson, 1987). Parents experience CP Workers as being uninterested in obtaining their viewpoint and in having little awareness of the effects that the CP Workers' own presence may have on their assessment of the parents and family. Because, however, only CP Workers, and not parents, report on the interaction between them, the "information" contained in the files favors the CP Worker's description of events. Conflict between CP Workers and parents is then described in terms of the parents' "problem" or pathology.

A major premise underlying child protection work is that the child's needs and interests must be paramount. As one CP Worker described it:

> " 'The child is your client.' That is supposed to make the scales fall from your eyes, somehow. It's supposed to give you focus, give you a way of working, but when it comes to the crunch, yes, by all means juggle things with the parents and whoever else you have to, but when it comes to the bottom line, you've got to do what is right for that kid."

In situations in which the parent and child have been in conflict with each other, the CP Worker's alliance with the child can be experienced by the parent as unfair and undermining. In describing how her daughter had run away after she had severely spanked her for stealing, Sally Travis reported:

"I felt that the Department was really against me, you know? . . . They were, or they appeared to be on her side, which was all right, but when it came to actually discussing the matter with me, no matter what I said to them it would seem to be wrong. They wouldn't consider it. Once they'd asked me a question, I'd answer that question, and if it didn't fit the way they thought I should feel, well, then it was wrong."

The conflict between parents and CP Workers over expectations for an adolescent is particularly acute when the family is an immigrant family from a non-English-speaking background. CP Workers may perceive the parents as abusive for physically punishing a girl who stayed out "late" on a date. To the CP Workers, the parents are unreasonable, and to the parents, the CP Workers are undermining their last vestiges of control.

This sense of always being in the wrong is particularly painful for those parents who had felt the Department to be on their side in the past. Lois Stevens had experienced child protection both from the perspective of a child and that of a single parent. Although she appreciated having the Department on her side as a child, she now felt betrayed that the CP Workers had turned against her as a parent:

"I think they should give both of them a chance. The parents and the children. Not just giving the children a chance. The parents are going through as much as everybody else is."

If the case involves an adolescent whose behavior is already difficult to control, the CP Worker's intervention is experienced as undermining the parents' authority and encouraging the child to act out, as one father described:

"They are more or less on the children's side, all the way. And the way I look at it, the bloody Department's standard today, the laws they're passing, I'd say in another 5 or 10 years and kids about 16 or 17 will be ordering their mother and father out of their own house and taking full control of it with the Department's backing up of it."

Parents' resistance to CP Workers is also connected to what they experience as an inherent "catch-22" created by the CP Worker's expectation that they acknowledge and "take responsibility" for the abuse. To "take responsibility" during the investigation process leaves parents in a quandary. To accept the label of "child abuser" is stigmatizing and humiliating. Such an admission can leave parents open to having the child removed and to facing legal prosecution. The more heatedly parents deny the allegations, however, the more likely they are to confirm the perception of CP Workers of themselves as "child abusers" because of their anger and their apparent failure to take responsibility for their behavior.

The dilemma faced by parents who are confronted with allegations was illustrated by Sandra Halleck, 28, mother of three young children. When her infant daughter was repeatedly hospitalized for whooping cough, Sandra confided in a hospital social worker that she felt tired, depleted, and overwhelmed with the demands of two toddlers at home. "Sometimes," she told the social worker, "I could just drown them." When Sandra next visited the hospital, she was confronted by two CP Workers concerning her "confidential" disclosure to the social worker. Believing she was being interrogated as a "child abuser," she countered by denying that she had ever been distressed:

> "They had about 20 accusations about things I'd said that I'd done to them! . . . Sure, I do say a lot of things, I did do a lot of them, but . . . the person who said that I said them has put in the punctuation marks and commas in the places where they shouldn't be. So I said, 'Look, I didn't do or say any of them so I want my kids back.' "

Feeling powerless to change their perception of her, Sandra argued heatedly with the CP Workers. The argument eventually culminated in her throwing a mug and then a chair at one of the Workers. This confirmed their perception of her as angry and out of control, and they felt justified in removing her children for a 3-month period despite having no physical evidence of harm to the children.

In order to have her children returned, Sandra believes that she was required to admit to being a "child abuser." In several meetings with CP Workers, she angrily denied any intention of hurting her children. As she recalled the events:

> "He [CP Worker] got me in and he said, 'When are you going to stop this bullshitting?' And I said, 'I don't have to put up with this. I'm not bullshittin' about anything.' He said, 'You're a child abuser. Why don't you admit it and get it all over and done with?' And I said, 'I'm not going to admit anything, nothing for you.' . . . He said, 'In other words you don't want your kids back.' I said, 'No, that's not true.' . . . I was thinking that if I admitted to being a child abuser, then they'd throw me into jail—forget about getting them back."

Finally realizing that the Department might be satisfied if she was to admit that she was desperate enough to have felt that she *could* have hurt her children, despite not having done so, Sandra finally discovered a way out of her dilemma.

"So, I went down and I said, 'Well, maybe I have had those feelings because, I mean, any mother feels at some stage she's going to kill 'em, but being able to control it as what counts.' And they said, 'Well, are you saying that you did it?' I didn't answer them and they just said, 'Well, OK, you can have Jessica back.' If I'd known this 6 weeks ago! Because I admitted to doing it—admitted to having the feelings!"

Little wonder that when Sandra was later referred to therapy by the Department, she was highly distrustful of all professionals.

Fathers accused of sexually abusing their children often face a similar "catch-22." In order to reunite with their families, CP authorities expect men to admit their guilt and take responsibility for the abuse. But if they do so, they are likely to face criminal charges and possible incarceration. They may be given legal advice to admit nothing. Consequently, very few men admit the abuse, take responsibility for their behavior, or talk in any depth with a therapist, who addresses their behavior and the context and values of which the abuse is a part. Therapy, if it does occur, is seen as only a brief stop on the way to the courtroom.[4]

COURT PROCEEDINGS

Court proceedings are seen by many therapists as having only a peripheral connection to the work of therapy. Court proceedings, however, may be enforcing the CP Worker's decision to send the parents to therapy, circumscribing the time for either therapy or removal of the children, and either creating for parents the leverage for change or, conversely, a sense of powerlessness and defeat. At the criminal level, the threat of imminent Court proceedings may bring a parent to therapy on the advice of a lawyer who thinks "it will look good," or, conversely, lock a parent into silence and avoidance of sessions for fear of providing evidence.

Many working-class parents lack even a basic understanding of legal discourse and feel overwhelmed and powerless in the face of Court proceedings. This is even more so if the parents are of a minority culture or non English speaking background. Parents are confused about what actually happens in court and unaware that the courtroom is a contest in

---

[4]The dilemmas involved in such situations have been successfully resolved through trial diversion programs, where men must admit their guilt but avoid prosecution so long as they and their family successfully undergo a 2-year treatment program. Unfortunately, the necessity for strict admission criteria for such programs, as well as their unavailability in less populated areas, means that for a great many men, they are not an option.

which their claims are matched against the claims of others. Few parents seek their own legal representation in the Children's Court. They are rarely assisted to do so and may actually be discouraged from doing so by their CP Workers. In those situations where the Court routinely provides a solicitor for parents, little use is made of this help. Parents perceive the outcome of the Court as a foregone conclusion over which the lawyer assigned to them has little influence. The difference between legal discourse and the discourse of these parents is often so great that the parents fail to provide the lawyer, and the lawyer fails to elicit, any information that would be useful to their case. As these two mothers described it:

"It's not much use. You know what the lawyer said? He said that they have a crackdown on this every now and again. He said, 'Oh well, they might pick up four families and might get lucky with one that it's happening to.' That's what he said."

"He didn't even turn up for the last court case. I didn't know until I got to court. He only saw me once. . . . I'd meet him at court, and he'd tell me before we went into court what was going to happen, and if I disapproved of anything, he couldn't seem to be able to do anything about it."

The Court is seen as an extension of or as being in collusion with the Department. CP Workers appear to be deciding both what information will be received by the Court and what the ultimate court decision will be. As one father speculated, "They have got it all tied up, because they've got that same judge." When a CP Worker takes charge of forwarding information to the court, reports that support the CP Worker's view of the situation are presented, and more positive assessments from other professionals may be included partially or not at all. Parents can conclude that the court outcome was decided at a departmental conference prior to the court proceedings.

"Like they tell you before you go to Court, they have a case conference. They tell you what's going to happen in Court and even a lawyer can't do that for you, and yet they can. They know what's going to happen to you at Court. They'll tell you if you're going to get off, and they try to tell you that 3 months is not too long to wait for your daughter to come back."

In states where a distinction exists between Criminal Courts and Children's Courts, this distinction is not always understood by the parents, resulting in some parents believing that they are on trial when the child's case is being heard in the Children's Court. Sandra described her terror over a 3-month period during which the Children's Court was determining whether to return her children. She believed she was being tried as a child abuser and could be sentenced to jail. Only 2 days before her children were returned, she learned through her lawyer that she had not "been on trial."

> "I didn't have the foggiest. They didn't let me know at all! . . . I was thinking I might end up in jail by tomorrow night, and that was really, really worrying me, because you know what happens to child abusers in jail, and I was thinking, 'Fancy going to jail for something I didn't do!' So I was a wreck a couple of days before each Court case."

Within such a confusing and intimidating context, the Court Order to attend therapy will usually be obeyed. Therapy, however, is likely to be perceived as an extension of the Department and the Courts. Therapy is something parents have to do to appease the Courts but is not something they want to do. Nor do they hold out any hope that therapy will be any less a place of judgment.

This chapter has overviewed the ways in which parents become clients of the CP Department and described the particular knots of interactional difficulties created by each of these paths of referral. Getting the parents' story of their experience with the Department prior to entering therapy allows us to understand, if not predict, their response to therapy and the extent of their motivation or resistance to changing family relationships. By creating a space in which the parents' experience of their referral to therapy can be given voice and received empathically and compassionately, a different context can be created in practice (see Chapter 6).

To understand why age and gender are significant factors in how parents respond to intervention, we must address another area that is a gap in the disease discourse of child abuse—family life in a working-class context. In the following chapter, we see how abuse is intimately connected with gendered relations and the material conditions of a family's existence. Parents who abuse children hold worldviews, often supported wholly or in part by cultural values and sanctions, that accept physical or sexual abuse as an option. Their worldviews are anchored in the discourses of the family and related notions of femininity, masculinity, heterosexuality, and parent–child relations.

CHAPTER FOUR

Working-Class Life
and the Family Ideal

THE overwhelming majority of child protection cases in the Western world consist of working-class families.[1] Whether, as those approaching child abuse from the disease discourse argue, this is simply a function of reporting patterns biased against the poor or whether it reflects, in fact, a higher incidence of child abuse among the working class, the net result is the same. Working-class families are the primary target of intervention.

This fact is significant for two reasons. First, the professionals who are required to intervene in these families are not working class. Whether or not a particular professional has moved up from the ranks of the working class, professionals occupy a very different social space than do these client families. The professional's space is socially privileged. Class and the professional's privileged position are rarely, if ever, addressed in the family therapy discourse (MacKinnon, 1993; McGoldrick, 1994).

---

[1]Although it is beyond the scope of this work to examine debates concerning the concept of class in any detail, it is important to acknowledge that the notion of class is vexed and is one that reflects little consensus among sociologists. I refer to as working class, first, all of those who rely on the wages of others and whose work is physically demanding, hard, frequently dirty, and, at times, dangerous, and who are often described as unskilled, semiskilled, and skilled manual workers; and, second, all those normally referred to as white-collar workers engaged in clerical and sales activities. I also include as working class those who rely on state support such as single-parent benefits, unemployment benefits, and social security income. I do not refer to as working class managers and professionals who work in both the private and public sector, whether or not they rely on the wages of others.

Professionally qualified immigrants may be engaged in working-class occupations in their new country because their skills are unrecognized or because racism prevents them from engaging in their area of skill. Their values and attitudes are likely to differ significantly from other working-class men and women, while many of their opportunities may be constrained in similar ways.

Working-class individuals have less control over their work situations and a lesser degree of power within interpersonal relationships in their work contexts than do professionals. Professionals are more able to set their own standards, determine in important ways the conditions of work and the rules under which that work should be undertaken. Professionals are able to exert power in the relationships that they establish with clients, patients, or consumers of the service that they provide (Western, 1983).

Professionals operate within a discourse that is valued in academic, bureaucratic, and political circles. The views and perspectives within that discourse are articulated both verbally through the audiovisual media and through the written word by people with status and position. The beliefs and experiences of the working class never reach such heights except on the rare occasion when an academic takes an interest in researching their perspectives. And even then, the researchers doing the speaking and the individuals being spoken about constitute two different groups.[2] The experiences of members of the working class who are of a less dominant racial, cultural, or ethnic group are even less well recognized. In this sense, working-class clients occupy the position of the professional's *others* (MacKinnon, 1993).

In feminist discourse, the "other" is that bit of ourselves that we are happy to disown and see in another person or group of people (Grosz, 1989). The *other* is socially and politically constructed as the subordinate group or individual. The *other* is our complement, existing in a relationship of subordination to our culturally defined dominance. Although the *other* is seen as "different," this difference is pseudo in that it is defined only within the terms of those who are dominant. Working-class clients do not have the opportunity to define themselves in their own terms and to have that definition recognized.

The second reason this fact is important to us is that the clinical discourses of child abuse imply but leave unstated a normative and ideal model against which families in treatment are judged. Although this ideal is shared by many other discourses and is one that impacts upon, and is embraced by, individuals from every level of the social strata, the options that exist for working-class men and women in attempting to live out this ideal are fewer that those for others of greater social status. I show later in this chapter that it is very often the attempts by working class men and women to fulfill this image of the ideal family that results in a restriction of their life chances and in a family form that has the ever-present potential for violence against women and children.

---

[2]This is inevitably the case with this book as well, despite my attempts to overcome some of these difficulties by including direct quotations or transcripts of the client's voice whenever possible.

The first section of this chapter overviews the discourse concerned with the family and contrasts the assumptions underlying the family ideal and the reality of family life in the 1990s. The second section presents an account of working-class family life, while drawing upon the perspectives of individuals whose families have experienced intervention by child protection authorities.

THE FAMILY IDEAL

Within clinical discourses concerning child abuse, "the family" is assumed to be a biological and natural, basic unit of society. All units other than those consisting of a heterosexual couple with their children thus fall into the category of "not family" and are to be considered in some way, deviant, broken, or illegitimate. Assumed to have always existed historically or, alternatively, to be the evolutionary outcome of human social progress, the family form itself, therefore, need not be questioned or explained by professionals. Rather, what does require explanation is all those sorts of arrangements that appear to fall short or outside of this definition and thus in some way reflect pathology or dysfunction. In this way, professional discourses are thus linked to the discursive formation of "the family," and the related preconceptions about femininity, masculinity, motherhood, and parent–child relations.

The "ideal" family is portrayed as white, middle-class, and of Anglo-Saxon origins. It consists of a father who, as breadwinner, works outside the home, a mother who takes responsibility for domestic duties, and children who go back and forth between home and school (Matthews, 1984). The family ideal is transmitted and reinforced through the media and dominant social institutions. It is transmitted from parents to children within family contexts through such things as role modeling of parents, prescriptions from parents of appropriate male and female behavior, and the unequal allocation of demands placed upon male and female children in the area of domestic labor.

Parents are perceived as failures when their children fail to conform to social norms in terms of health, behavior, or academic success. The burden of this failure, however, does not fall equally on the shoulders of both men and women. Because it is seen as women's responsibility to manage and care for the children, it is mothers who are subject to surveillance and judgment from themselves, the community, and the state (Matthews, 1984). It is the question of the mother's "goodness" that lies at the heart of the state's deliberation concerning whether parents are determined to be "fit" (Wilkinson, 1987).

The positions of "father" and "mother" carry with them ideal attributes concerning masculinity and femininity, which parents must fulfill to meet the conditions of the ideal family. Deviations from attaining these ideals are viewed as a failure, and failure, as a fault (Wilkinson, 1987). The discursive formation concerning the family is comprised of a set of interrelated assumptions:

1. *Motherhood is natural and normal and provides ultimate fulfillment for women.* To be perceived as mature, balanced, self-fulfilled adults, it is necessary for women to become mothers (Wearing, 1984; Braverman, 1989).

2. *The ideal mother is heterosexual, monogamous, and legally married.* A good woman attaches herself to a man, restricts her sexuality to the fulfillment of his needs, and remains within the institution of marriage. Women fall from this ideal through pregnancy out of wedlock, lesbianism, prostitution, promiscuity, or divorce (Matthews, 1984).

3. *A good mother is willing to sacrifice her own needs for those of her children.* She is unselfish, puts her children's needs first, and willingly assumes total responsibility for child care.

4. *Because women are the biological bearers of children, child care and domestic labor are naturally their job.* This division of labor is considered fair because it is perceived as balanced by men's participation in the paid workforce and responsibility for the financial support of the family (Goode, 1982).

5. *Masculinity is defined in terms of a man's occupational success and his ability to provide a home for his family and education for his children.* The worth of a man is based upon his individual ability, and his lack of success in the world results from a lack of this ability. From this perspective, when a man fails to achieve as much as his neighbor, he can only hold himself to blame.

6. *Physical prowess reflects the degree of a man's masculinity.* Masculinity is defined through the male body in terms of strength, aggression, and sexuality. Images of ideal masculinity are constructed and promoted most systematically through competitive sport. Male schoolchildren are encouraged to remain engaged in competitive sports and to regard their success as deeply important (Connell, 1987, p. 85).

7. *It is natural for men to be dominant in male–female relationships.* Because physical prowess reflects masculinity, a woman who is younger, smaller, and deferent to a man confirms his sense of himself as masculine. On the other hand, expressing emotional vulnerability, or needs for dependence or nurturance, defines a man as weak and unmasculine. Expressions of vulnerability are

to be avoided unless they can be expressed through sexual means.

8. *Male sex drive requires a regular outlet, and it is the responsibility of women in marriage to service and contain male sexual needs.* Men's "need" for intercourse is seen as normal and functional, whereas a woman's apparent lack of interest in intercourse is seen as abnormal or dysfunctional (James & MacKinnon, 1990; Hare-Mustin, 1994).

9. *Parents have the right and duty to socialize children into "being good."* Parents are responsible for instilling within their children values concerning punctuality, regularity, diligence, thrift, sobriety, standard language, uniform dress, patriotism, and respect for authority (Matthews, 1984; van Krieken, 1986).

It has been through the intersection of a number of social developments that the ideal of the family has evolved (Luepnitz, 1988; Aries, 1962; Gilding, 1991). These include, first, the change in the late 18th century in discourses concerning the value of children and the place of women as mothers. Second, paid work became separated from domestic labor and thus the spheres in which men and women circulated day to day became separate. Men became absent from the daily experiences of women and children. Third, there was a great proliferation of experts who advanced knowledge and actively intervened in child care on medical and educational fronts. Fourth, there was a reduction of households from large and changing networks of kin and, in some classes, servants, to households consisting primarily of nuclear families whose homes were often situated some distance from the father's work location (Matthews, 1984; Gilding, 1991).

The intersection of these particular developments led to the proliferation of "families" in the 1950s and 1960s and the baby boom following World War II. This was soon followed by an expansion of interest in "the family" by the behavioral sciences, including social work, psychology, and sociology, and the emergence of the field of family therapy (Gilding, 1991). The research and literature in these areas primarily reflected white, middle-class, heterosexual couples with children (Graham, 1992; Clulow, 1993).

The optimistic ideal of "the family" stands in sharp contrast to the suffering that is often experienced within families:

1. Rather than the fulfillment expected in marriage, women may find themselves raped, beaten, and verbally abused by their husbands. Although escape from unhappy or violent marriages is easier and less stigmatizing than it once was, economic depend-

ence and psychological commitment keep many women in abusive relationships for years (Strube & Barbour, 1983).

2. Rather than the care and protection expected from within their
families, children may be sexually assaulted by male adult family
members, very often their father.

3. Rather than the ultimate fulfillment expected in motherhood,
traditional gender arrangements leave many women who are
caring for children, alone, isolated and depressed.

4. Parents may physically assault children as a means of achieving
their compliance. A major contributing factor to the high level
of parent–child violence is the normative acceptability of hitting
one's children (Gelles & Straus, 1987). The law enshrines the
right of parents to use physical force by distinguishing between
assaults against children by a parent and assaults against adults by
adults (Scutt, 1983).

Family life in the 1990s also varies considerably from that of family
life during the 1950s and 1960s in the following major ways:

1. Fewer families in Western countries fit the image of a white,
Anglo-Saxon, middle-class family with two biological parents and
children. Immigration to Western countries, particularly from
Asia, has contributed to a multi-cultural landscape (Graham,
1992; Clulow, 1993). In the United States, the prevalence of racial
and Hispanic minorities has increased at a much higher rate than
those of non-Hispanic whites. The traditional family will continue to become less prevalent in Western countries as there is an
increasing number of different types in families including, but not
limited to, African American, Hispanic, single-parent, and stepparent families (Fine, 1993; McGill, 1992).

2. There is a much higher rate of single parenthood, divorce, and
remarriage. The liberalization of divorce laws and increased state
support for single parents have provided hitherto unknown options for women. Greater social tolerance has also resulted in a
significant rise in families headed by gay and lesbian parents
(Alpert, 1988; Weston, 1991).

3. The majority of women reenter the workforce during their married life. For working-class families, this is often a necessity if they
are to buy their own home. Many women carry a double load of
paid and unpaid labor.

4. Whether or not it ever was, the gendered division of labor is no
longer "different but equal." No financial necessity has compelled
men to take up an equitable share of unpaid domestic labor in the
manner in which women have been compelled to take paid labor.

Time budget studies show that marriage doubles women's unpaid labor while decreasing men's already low level of indoor work and only mildly increasing outdoor tasks (Bittman, 1991).

5. There is considerable evidence that despite the tendency to treat individuals within different types of families as homogeneous, they are, in fact, heterogeneous and diverse (Fine, 1993).

Although the family ideal impacts upon individuals of all social strata, the options available in living out this ideal are affected by income, ethnicity, and class:

1. Social arrangements based on racial differences privilege whites and exclude people of color from access to power and resources, all the while blaming them for their failure (Pinderhughes, 1989). Low-income African Americans and Australian Aborigines, for example, must deal with inadequate community services, poor housing, and chronic unemployment. African Americans, Asian Americans, Latinos, Native Americans, and women of color, in particular, are disproportionately represented in the lowest economic groups and in occupations with the poorest pay (Graham, 1992).

2. Migration to Western countries may empower women, who benefit from the new country's liberalized values and protective laws. Their male partners, however, accustomed to a dominant position, may feel disempowered both within the family and in the job market.

3. Greater occupational success for men means that the experience of power and the struggle to prove themselves against other men can be transferred into the symbolic realm of money and occupational achievements.

4. For women, greater income increases the ability to buy the services of other women, thus enabling the tasks of child rearing and domestic labor to be undertaken with less personal effort, perhaps allowing for greater achievement in the public world. Although the options afforded to members of the upper social strata do not make them immune from violence, the struggles faced by them are different than those faced by working-class families.

5. Access to further education opens the door to competing discourses through which individuals can perceive opportunities for constructing themselves differently. This is the case, for example, when women encounter feminist ideas as part of their university courses.

The following section examines how the interaction of family, school, and work reproduces working class culture and how the ideal of the family impacts upon working-class men and women in a manner that results in a restriction of their life chances.

WORKING-CLASS LIFE

The account of working-class life that follows is written largely from the perspective of women.[3] This is because women are more likely to become the clients of child protection services or of therapists, whether or not they are perceived as being the alleged abusers (Corby, 1993; Langeland & Dijkstra, 1995). In part, this reflects the high proportion of single-parent women, a result of women separating from their husbands in order to escape violence or after a child discloses sexual abuse. Despite the frequency with which men are the alleged abusers, women are more likely than men to have ongoing contact with either CP Workers or therapists. CP Workers are more able to engage women than men in treatment, women are more likely to ask for help, and women are often more available during office hours. Where there is insufficient evidence to "establish a case" against a suspected abuser, CP Workers' focus and the push into therapy generally remain on the "primary caregiver"—the mother.

I have chosen to present an account of family contexts in chronological order, ranging from working-class schooling, independence and escaping from home, through to marriage and then to escaping from marriage and parenting alone. I then examine the ideology of control and how it informs parents' understandings of their responsibility for and their relationship to their children.

Working-Class Schooling

The peer and school cultures of working-class children is the seed of development of masculinity and femininity. It is through the rejection of values concerned with achievement and compliance with authority that

---

[3]Quotations in this section are drawn from the research project. The descriptions and conceptualizations of family life are drawn from both my research and other research sources in Australia and the United States. These studies describe working-class life in the two countries similarly. None of these studies, however, privileges race or ethnicity. I thus suspect there will be many similarities and some differences to the descriptions presented here among specific ethnic or cultural groups. In a context of racism, the differences seen in minority racial groups may be more appropriately conceptualized as racial or cultural, rather than class issues (Boyd-Franklin, 1989).

boys and girls turn to traditional notions of masculinity and femininity and in doing so restrict their future life options (Sennett & Cobb, 1972; McRobbie, 1978; Donaldson, 1991; Samuel, 1983). In working-class schools, children learn a lifelong lesson: Individual worth is based upon individual ability, and lack of success in the world results from a lack of this ability. In the large, working-class classroom, teachers selectively recognize and reinforce the few students who appear to have a particular ability to "get ahead" and "make something of themselves." With such recognition, these children tend to improve their performance and become increasingly competent in contrast to other students. By maintaining school values, these "chosen few" pay the price of peer rejection and loneliness, which reinforces their dedication to their areas of competence. These are the few who continue through to tertiary education and ultimately enter occupations with professional status (Sennett & Cobb, 1972). As one mother described:

> "That is how you brought up kids in those days. They were locked in the closet, beaten up on a regular basis, ignored, not spoken to. That was just how you brought up children, and somehow or other, most of them came through it quite adequately, so that's how we were brought up. . . . I was living my life to get what was necessary to get me out of that house, that country town, educated and away. That's what I did. . . . What got me out of that situation was the fact that I'm smart, and that sounds awful, but the fact that I'm intelligent was good at school, enabled me, instead of being kicked out of home and school at 14, like everyone else was, to get a scholarship to go on to fifth year. That was the final year. Then other scholarships to go on to university, and that's how I got out. . . . "

In contrast, the many unrecognized students perceive their lack of recognition and success as a consequence of their lack of ability and suffer a loss of self-esteem and dignity. Their struggle to overcome this sense of inadequacy, failure, and loss of dignity generates a process of resistance on the part of some children, culminating in a counterculture defined by its opposition to school rules and expectations. Boys reject the school and the "goody goodies" who comply with its rules. A counterculture of male dignity springs forth, through which success is defined in terms of toughness and strength. Behavior such as smoking, drinking, taking drugs, having sex, using pornography, and truancy is encouraged and applauded (Donaldson, 1991; Sennett & Cobb, 1972). The force and skill involved in competitive sports is one means by which masculinity becomes a statement embodied through postures and muscle tensions, ultimately affecting the interaction between men and women, and between men of greater and lesser prowess. This is one of the main ways in which the power of men becomes "naturalized" (Connell, 1987, p. 85).

Manual labor becomes associated with social superiority and masculinity, connoting strength, activity, hardness, danger, difficulty, and courage. Mental labor, in contrast, is experienced as connoting social inferiority and femininity. Boys are thus attracted to jobs that require little education and make use of the strength of their bodies. Such work generates a preoccupation with their bodies and a concern with physical strength (Donaldson, 1991).

Rejecting school values of achievement and compliance takes girls along a different but complementary path. Female peer groups center around heterosexuality and stereotypic views of femininity that emphasize fashion and beauty. Girls perceive marriage and family life as their true vocations and work as a stopgap before marriage (McRobbie, 1978; Burns, 1986). Their options for work are few, and most will settle for unskilled jobs with minimal wages in such traditional areas as assembly, sales and clerical work, or work as receptionists, typists, and secretaries.

Independence and Escaping from Home

Although young men turn to work for the sense of independence and success that school denied them, manual work offers little recognition or autonomy. Constant orders and surveillance are experienced as depersonalizing and infantilizing. Rather than attribute their unhappiness to the nature of their jobs, however, they perceive their failure to enjoy work as confirmation that there is indeed something wrong with themselves. The expression of their unhappiness must also be contained. Those who persist with a "bad attitude" may lose their jobs or find themselves in situations created to "break their spirit." Boredom and frustration results in organized militancy, practical joking, and transference of the desire to hit back physically into areas where little challenge or contestation is expected (Donaldson, 1991). For men of a racial or ethnic minority, prospects for dependable work are often limited despite the visible affluence of the country. The last to be hired and the first to be fired, they are left feeling publicly humiliated (Almeida, Woods, Messineo, Font, & Heer, 1994).

For both young men and women, the experiences within (often) authoritarian families, demeaning school environments, and ultimately unsatisfying work leaves a yearning to establish themselves as independent persons. Marriage is perceived to be a means to this end. Young women on minimal wages find it difficult to support themselves apart from their families of origin unless they marry. For boys, the prospect of marriage offers a haven from the heartless world of work and other men, a place where they might reveal their "real" selves, express their needs, loneliness and fears, as well as have their domestic needs anticipated and fulfilled.

The ideal of the family and motherhood is willingly embraced by working-class girls not only because it is a means of rejecting school culture but also because the material constraints of working-class life leave girls to conclude that marriage and motherhood is a preferred option. A career of motherhood compares favorably to the mindless and powerless positions that are generally available to working-class women in the labor force. Partnership with a man allows girls access to greater financial means than would be available through the low-paid work available to women (Donaldson, 1991). Children allow women to create the experience of an intense emotional relationship, the type of relationship that they may seek with men but which, due to the dictates of "masculinity" and work culture, men most frequently fail to meet (Chodorow, 1978).

Perhaps most important, the "choice" of marriage and motherhood for most working-class girls is not experienced as any choice at all. They are kept in place on the one hand by economic imperatives and on the other by the social stigma of women unattached to men. They are deprived of any other perspective either through the media or their own social network of women as "passionate comrades, life partners, coworkers, lovers, tribe" (Rich, 1980). Heterosexuality is a compulsory way of life, one never questioned, one experienced as "only natural" (Kitzinger, 1987).

Some girls are sidetracked from their goal of marriage by an overwhelming desire to escape from home. Within a few years, these young women in their late teens and early 20s will become clients of the CP Department. They leave home at an early age, a move precipitated by the separation of their parents or an attempt to escape violence or sexual abuse. Witnessing their father's violence, directed at themselves or their mother, they learn about using force as a way of obtaining compliance. As these two young women described it:

"Dad used to drink, come home and bash Mum, then you'd stick up for Mum and you got bashed up. . . . Every second night, from Thursday to Monday, you could guarantee that Dad would be drunk at night and that Mum would get bashed. . . . Dad would do it and I used to do it at school. If I had the shits with anyone, if I had the shits with you, I'd go and smack you. . . . If you had an excuse, that's what you did, you bashed them."

"I ran away from home because Dad used to get real cranky and would chuck a pitchfork at me or something like that. . . . They used to want to get rid of me and all that. They threatened to put me in a home, but I just didn't let it get to me. . . . At one stage he was getting really dirty and wanting me to do these really dirty things, and I just wouldn't have it. And I tried never to be alone with him again."

The distrust of authority that they learned within the home is compounded by the refusal or inability of authorities outside the family to offer protection from their fathers' violence:

"The cops won't do anything about that. You know he was really strangling her . . . but they weren't going to do anything about it because it was a 'domestic argument.' "

"Dad gave me a hiding once, when I was a kid. And I went to school and the teacher asked me where the marks came from and I wouldn't tell them. And they said, you know, 'We can report your father for this.' . . . I just said, I don't know what I said, but I got out of it. . . . If I didn't, I would have copped another hiding."

Pregnancy for these women is a way of exiting the home situation and bringing adolescence to an abrupt halt. Although unplanned and "accidental," the idea of having a child is often welcomed, and there is little consideration of terminating the pregnancy. The work and skills entailed in motherhood, however, demands more from them than they anticipate, as these three women explained:

"No, I didn't really feel up to it. I wanted to be a mother but I didn't know how. That was the main problem when I was young, when I was 17. That's normal, eh? . . . I was just too confused then. I suppose I knew that if I kept living my life the way I was that I was going to have a baby, but I didn't do anything to stop it, did I? I didn't really care. I didn't decide. I just didn't think about it. I put it out of my mind. . . . I didn't want an abortion. Well, Mum never believed in abortion, so I didn't. I was a bit young to have me own set of ideas or anything."

"When I was a kid, I had a few hassles and left home when I was 15 and all that stuff, you know, I just wandered around. . . . I was 17 or 18 . The next thing I was pregnant, I had Sandy, and what else, then I had a baby that died. . . . I didn't know anything about Sandy. I had no idea. I laugh at it now but I was so dumb! . . . She was an accident. Yeah, I hated kids. I thought I'm never going to have kids. I'm never going to get married, and I hate the little brats. I remember when I found out I was pregnant, I was totally unprepared for it. . . . I could have had it [an abortion]. I just didn't want it. Mum tried to talk me into it ... but I said I could handle the world if it blew up at the time.... I don't believe in abortions. Even though I don't go to church, I'm a very religious person."

"I look back now and I was very young, not real young, I was 19, like I'd been nowhere and done nothing and I'd had a hell of a bloody life, and like here I am with the baby, what am I going to do? He was a drunk, he always wanted to go out. He wouldn't want to take me out because of the way I used to go on. I used to get kicked out of pubs even then."

When they learn of the pregnancy, they want the baby, perceiving it as "something to be proud of," something that, for once, would be their very own. While knowing little about the practicalities of caring for a baby, they anticipate becoming "perfect mothers":

"I was in the waiting room and he said, 'Yeah, you know you're pregnant.' And I was so shocked to think I was pregnant, you know, and then it dawned on me that I was going to have this baby. I was going to have somethink [sic] that belonged to me. It was mine! ... I didn't care if it was a boy or a girl. It was something that I had. ... It was my baby, and I could love him and he would love me, you know, and all that. I had so many wonderful things planned. I was going to be the perfect mother. Mind you, I knew nothing about kids, but I was going to be the perfect mother and everything, but things didn't work out that way."

Young mothers describe the most difficult aspects of mothering as, first, being tied down, constantly in demand, lacking in freedom, privacy, and the ability to plan ahead or complete tasks; and, second, the child's disobedience, whining, answering back, cheekiness, temper tantrums, and the discipline involved (Wearing, 1984). Having underestimated the demands of caring for infants and young children, they cannot turn to the fractured relationships of their families of origin for support. On their own or in relationships with men who are unreliable and often violent, they talk about not coping and their desperate need for a break from the children:

"I'd been sick. I'd been stuck in the house all the time. He would go out and I was just stuck with the baby all the time, day in and day out, which wasn't good for me because I wasn't well to start with."

"I did need help actually, I needed a break from the kids, right? So I went around to all the so-called social workers and asked if I could have someone mind the kids for a weekend every now and again just to give me a break, because I was by myself. The children's father was dead. I was 18 when I had the two little ones. It was a bit tough. . . . I asked for help and they sort of brushed me off, and they thought I just wanted a good time, and a few months later I started to have a nervous breakdown and they suggested to have the kids fostered, and I didn't want that. After about a year, I ended up getting them fostered."

Whereas the relationship between the mother and her male partner often begins with an intense bonding and optimism, the presence of a child, particularly an infant, strains their relationship, frequently leading to mutual disappointment and feelings of anger and exploitation. The birth of the child monumentally increases the amount of work for the woman, leaving her tired and less available for her male partner. His lack of support, emotionally and with domestic labor, increases her resentment. He feels rejected, exploited for the income he provides, and if unemployed, criticized for his lack of contribution. In this context, infants receive injuries, many of them serious. How the injuries occur is often unclear to the mother, but in most cases they are attributable to her partner. When children are older, the situation is less overwhelming but still stressful. Children frequently reject new stepfathers, and stepfathers in turn perceived the children as being unruly and out of control. Relationships between these young women and their partners seldom last.

Finding it difficult to manage the demands of what becomes a young family of two or three children, some of these young mothers become what professionals call careless or negligent, at times resorting to harsh physical discipline or "lashing out." At some stage, many of these young mothers either relinquish or involuntarily lose their children to foster care for a period of time. Once caught in this life situation, options for these young women are few. With little emotional or practical support, no financial backing or promise of inheritance from their own families, little education, few marketable skills, and the dependence of young children, their chances of improving their material lot in life are small. A few may turn to prostitution in order to improve their standard of living and to provide more materially for their children. Others look to attach themselves to another man.

Black Families

Adolescent parenthood for African Americans may not be the negative experience it is for many others. Although motherhood is also an important part of the role image for African American women, it is not presumed that the mother will care for the child on her own. Rather, the majority of black children born out of wedlock are cared for within extended family networks (Boyd-Franklin, 1989) in which the primary "parent" is often the child's maternal grandmother.

Many grandmothers in African American families are, in fact, fairly youthful and have had their own children during their teenage years. They were raised as siblings to their own children and now, in turn, become the "mother" to their grandchildren. Thus, as they age, these women often experience an increase rather than a decrease in family responsibilities (Boyd-Franklin, 1989). The grandmothers remain a major power in extended families even if the mother is, herself, the primary caretaker.

Although this arrangement often works successfully when the children are young, problems may emerge later when the mother wants to resume primary care of her adolescent child. Such transitions are difficult, because the mother has to displace her own mother as the central authority and become a "mother" to a child who has perceived her in the role of a sibling (Boyd-Franklin, 1989).

Marriage and Family Life

For the working-class man, marriage offers a refuge from the world of work, a separate sphere in which the man believes he can be himself. Sexuality is one of the few areas in which working-class men can develop and express themselves. In sex, "male workers have increasingly sought solace, release and an assertion of power. . . . Sex is often the one way a man's emotional control is shaken, where he can contact and express his deeper feelings" (Donaldson, 1991, p. 26). The attachment to one woman, however, and the significance attached to sexuality, leaves men precariously dependent on their wives and fearful of their potential for infidelity, which could transmit to another man their wives' secret knowledge of their deeper selves (Donaldson, 1991).

On the other hand, marriage offers another opportunity for men to experience themselves as failures. If he is not to fail, a working-class man must obtain a steady job, education for the children, a home for the family, and freedom from the threat of poverty (Kleinberg, 1979). For some, however, employment is, at best, cyclical, at the mercy of the economic up- and downturns. For working-class men of color, prospects for dependable work are always only tenuous and the humiliation of chronic unemployment always threatening (Almeida et al., 1994). In contrasting themselves to other men, working-class men perceive themselves, to some degree or other, as having failed. Believing they had an "equal go" at school, they can only attribute this failure to their own lack of merit and ability. Those who succeed do so because they deserve to, work harder, try harder, are brighter or more diligent. "The question of their masculinity is constantly confronting them, constantly being tested, constantly being found inadequate" (Donaldson, 1991, p. 30). Masculinity therefore remains a tenuous and ever-threatened achievement.

Marriage and family responsibilities thus bind men more closely to paid labor. In their attempt to derive some sense of meaning and dignity from unsatisfying work, working-class men come to perceive work as a sacrifice for their families, an effort exerted in the hopes that their children can become more successful than they themselves and thus experience greater rewards in the work world. Children's education becomes highly valued. In making such a sacrifice, however, men can come to perceive the family as an imposition, a millstone, an impediment to an imaginary better future. Sacrificing himself so that his children *will not be like himself*, he denigrates himself before other family members. Children may perceive fathers' sacrifices as manipulative or, alternatively, may disappoint their fathers by failure to live up to their expectations (Sennett & Cobb, 1972; Donaldson, 1991). Last, the investment of time that work requires leaves men peripheral and excluded from the intensity of the mother–child relationships at home (James & McIntyre, 1982).

On the one hand, the relationship between men and women in the family–household is based upon the perceived complementarity of their needs. For both, it promises an escape from the control, frequently patriarchal, of the family of origin and initiation into independence and autonomy. For her, it promises the career of motherhood, a career that is perceived to offer greater autonomy and satisfaction than the boring, low paid, low-status jobs for women in the workplace. It also rescues her from the stigma of the unmarried woman and initiates her into the network of other wives and mothers. For him, it promises a refuge from the world of men and work, where he may have his masculinity validated and confirmed. In the family–household, he may exert the influence he sees himself lacking at work. His children offer the hope of making meaning of otherwise meaningless work, and in the context of an ongoing sexual relationship with a woman, he might explore and express his vulnerability, a part of him repressed in all other contexts.

Although, no doubt, the family–household fulfills these promises for many working-class men and women, its success for others at different life stages is, at most, tenuous (Rubin, 1992). Women may come to feel trapped by constant child care, which is demanding, exhausting, and often boring. Social isolation—parenting alone or inadequate support from friends, kin, or partner—may unbalance an already precarious ability to cope.

Few women can avoid reentering the workforce at some stage of their lives. Yet, the double load of organizing and maintaining a household while engaged in paid work is exceedingly stressful, tiring, and unromantic, leaving little energy for the emotional and sexual nurturance expected by the husband. Working class women become disillusioned with the unequal exchange on which the family–household is based (Burns, 1986). Her burden of never-ending domestic labor, the hours she spends working while he drinks, sleeps, or plays sports, or his failure to maintain work or bring home adequate income, erodes her sense of fairness in the arrangement. She may respond by curtailing emotional and sexual services, by criticizing what he perceives as aspects of his masculinity, and by refusing the deference he believes to be his lot. In doing so, he perceives her as provoking his anger, his fear, and, in some cases, his violence (Donaldson, 1991). He may assert, perhaps with his fists, what he believes to be his rights to a well-cared-for home, undemanding children, and sexual and emotional access.

The second group of parents to become clients of the Department are in their 30s and 40s, married one or more times, and currently in a marriage of several years duration. Although these parents unite against a perceived threat from outsiders, marriages are often unhappy, particularly for the women. The husband's dominant position is established early on in the marriage, often through violence and intimidation.

For some women, physical abuse is a constant feature of their relationship, as one woman described her 14-year marriage:

> "I just couldn't possibly remember just how many times I thought this was my last breath, because he was choking me, and how he ever let go in time, I don't know. He smashed things. You just had to put one word wrong and his foot would go through a door, his fist would go through a cupboard or a wall. It was terrible . . . on average, once a week for the best part of our marriage."

For others, the husband's violence is less consistent, emerging from time to time or in particular circumstances. The threat of his violence is, nevertheless, enough to maintain his domination:

> "My husband was a quietly threatening sort of person . . . who dominated everyone by his temper and by manipulation. . . . His way of ruling the house was by fear, that if you don't do as you're told there'll be trouble. And what he used to do was get drunk and then it would be miserable for everybody, because he was a very violent drunk."

Other women avoid abuse by adopting a subservient position to their husbands, fearing that standing up to him could elicit a violent attack.

The threat of violence is seen to be very real. At some stage early in their marriage, the husband was violent, and the woman believes that it is only through appeasing him that his violence remains under control:

> "Well, we really must do what he wants, not that we're particularly happy about everything. . . . I'm probably too weak. My mother-in-law tells me I should stand up to him more, but he'll yell at me. . . . He can be sort of violent. I don't mean hitting me or anything like that, but just by yelling. . . . He kicked me in the backside once, in temper, when I was 7 months pregnant. . . . In fact, he used to punch me in the stomach saying, 'I'm going to mug this bloody kid.' . . . He'll yell, and so on, and really looks fierce and scares me, and I suppose scares the kids too a bit at times."

Even if his wife does "her jobs" well, however, he may feel excluded and rejected by, first, the imbalance of his, compared to her, emotional dependence on their relationship and, second, by the intensity of her relationship with the children. He may turn against the children physically, perhaps in the name of discipline, or he may turn to one of his children and engage her or him into a secretive and destructive relationship of sexual exploitation.

Few mothers describe affection between fathers and children. The father's involvement with the children is frequently limited to controlling their behavior and asserting a feared and authoritative presence. Fear of the father frequently solidifies a coalition between the mother and children in their attempts to protect themselves from him:

> "He is far too quick-tempered. You know, he can't talk to a kid, he has to yell, for some reason, I don't know. But with me, I talk to 'em, I don't yell at 'em, and I find that's the difference between him and I. . . . Those kids are turning into a nervous wreck. I can't even raise my hand to scratch my head like that without my kids jumping. . . . These kids are either going to end up in a hospital as nervous wrecks or they're going to end up in a mental home being so scared of their father. . . . The kids are always ducking as if I'm going to, you know, throw it at them or something."

> "I've had my kids turn around and say to me, 'Mummy I hate my father, I'm scared of him. Why can't you get rid of him?' And I've just had to turn around and say to 'em, 'Look, I can't, I married your father and it's, you know, I've got to try and bear with him.' You know, I've turned around and told them, 'Look, I'm going to try and make him better if I can.' "

"He never used to belt my son around, but when he hit him, he always hit on the head, across the face and head. He thinks it's soft, but it's not, it's hard, and you could never get through his head that it's really hurting. . . . So my son was always the one who was copping the slaps and my daughter would get away with everything, and my son used to always turn to me and my husband used to go off about that, because he used to say it was making him a sissy because he would turn to me. Because we were close, he was closer to me because he couldn't get close to him. You know, there was no affection or anything. He wouldn't show Jamie affection or anything."

"The boys never wanted to be alone with him even when we were still married. They were only left once alone with him overnight in all that amount of time. When my mother was operated on for cancer, when I came back the next morning, the kids came running up to me and cuddling me and all."

"I think we'd all be happier without him. I really do. I'm not trying to be horrible. Yes, probably he does intimidate us a lot. Yes, he probably can't see it at all because he doesn't want to. But yeah, we would probably be happier."

Although these women may be perceived by professionals as collusive with their husband's mistreatment of the children, the mothers themselves believe they can do little to halt the father's harsh treatment of their children. As one recently separated mother commented, "If I tried to do anything I would have copped it as much as my son did, if not more. How could I stop it? If I say the wrong thing, I get my head smashed in."

The intense involvement of women with children and the peripheral nature of the father's involvement is in part an artifact of the traditional family form that locates women within the domestic sphere and men in the public sphere. For men whose life histories and work contexts sensitized them to issues of rejection and humiliation, the division of family relationships in this manner feeds their perception of being excluded and unwanted. One father who said he worked two jobs as a manual laborer to afford to buy his wife and four children a family home, described how extended hours away from his wife and children increased his sense of vulnerability to rejection:

"When I started working the second job, I had too much time on me own, away from the family, and I was wondering if er, if she, I didn't think she would have another relationship. I was working about 20 hours on the second job, about 60 hours altogether. [*And that was when you started getting the idea that she didn't love you?*] Yeah, yeah. It started to hit very hard, and got very close inside me. I was shutting down me feelings, and I didn't give a hang."

Locked into work made meaningful only by sacrifice for the family yet perceiving his wife and children as aligned against him, and himself as excluded from the only emotionally sustaining relationship he has, violence or sexual abuse may be the father's solution to his feelings of humiliation, hurt, fear of loss, and desire to be included and belong. But these needs are disguised and dressed in the acceptably masculine desire for control and demand for respect. His perception of his sacrifices for the family justify (to him) his right to expect the family to act as he wishes. In the end, however, the accumulated incidents of violence or the disclosure of sexual abuse lead to his increased isolation and deepen his feelings of rejection. As one father described:

"I learned to growl at an early age, put people on guard. I'm not really a vicious person, but I found that if I could bellow down enough, people would say, 'Oh,' and then back off. But most of the time I probably was as big a coward as ... (*laughs*). But I learned from an early age that if I sort of made threats with Katherine, or threats with the family, I felt as if I was in control. .... Because, you know, people would be frightened of me, oh, not exactly frightened of me, but they'd respect me. I thought they'd respect me, and I was hoping they wouldn't hurt me, as a protection, you know? ... I was always frightened of getting hit, for some reason. ... But I think what it was, if I could say, 'I'll punch your head in,' or offer some defense of violence, people would back off, and I think it was wearing very thin with a lot of people. It wasn't a defense at all. I think people used to think, 'I can't be bothered with him,' and walk away ... and that would make me really angry then."

The threat of the father's violence is often sufficient to ensure his control over the children's behavior. The mother's coalition with the children, however, whether due to the father's violence or his emotional or physical absence, means that she holds less authority with them and correspondingly has greater difficulty managing their behavior. To maintain her closeness with them, she either fails to set limits for their behavior, does so inconsistently, or periodically indulges them. When she becomes increasingly exasperated with their behavior, she has two choices: to align with the father and make use of the authority he commands, or attempt to regain some measure of authority herself, a difficult task under the circumstances and one accomplished most easily through physical means.

For some mothers, however, even physical force does not accomplish the desired end of being in control of the children. The mother's inconsistent, sometimes hard, sometimes soft approach fuels the children's rebellion. As the children became older the "contest of wills" between them becomes more frequent. Situations escalated into episodes in which, blinded by a sense of helplessness and rage, mothers experience few options other than what some called "bashing" their children. The children, in turn, confused and angered by their mother's inconsistency and betrayal, become harder, more withdrawn, more rejecting, ultimately becoming the sort of children that parents say "invite abuse."

The children's perception of the mother's weak position in the marriage and the mother's diminishing ability to control the children as they grow older ultimately contributes to a relationship between mothers and children in which the children show little respect for her or what she says. This is particularly so with male children who have grown up in a family and cultural context that supports male dominance and violence. "Boys need a father," say these mothers, who describe how their sons would not listen to mothers whose authority they do not accept. One mother, for example, who tried several times to separate from her husband, who drank heavily and beat her frequently, said she "always went back" because she found it too difficult to cope on limited financial resources and deal with five boys who "had no respect" for her and had become increasingly like their father in behavior.

Escaping from Marriage and Parenting Alone

Separation does not initially appear to be a solution to the husband's violence. In separating from abusive husbands, women sometimes face further violence or threats and feel their lives are constrained with fear:

> "He is so *angry* with me, he is so *angry*. If there ever was domestic violence, he is the one. I fear for my life, I really do, I really fear for my life. . . . I've been in hospital twice. Fractured jaw bone, perforated ear drums. Last Wednesday, he hit me again. I had to take out an assault charge and a restraining order."

> "I was terrified. At one stage we were living in darkness, virtually. We had the TV on at night but we had all the lights turned off, and we'd have blankets over the windows so there'd be no light from the TV showing. We'd have it on quiet, wouldn't let the kids out, had

to walk them to and from school. We were just living in fear because Bob was going around making all these threats how he put me in hospital and how he'd come and grab the kids and take off with them. He was just making all these threats, because I was standing up to him and he hated that. He cannot stand me standing up to him."

Those who have attempted separation are fearful of its emotional and material consequences, in particular, single parenthood and poverty:

"I mean, I'd been separated before, and I knew how tough it is, and that's very hard when you're on your own. I'd been separated when he'd been in jail and the kids had been little. I'd been through some pretty awful experiences then. When the kids were very little, my mum refused to have me home any more because she said it was time to stand on my own two feet. And Jeanie was only 2 weeks old and Jack was only 2 at the time."

"I went to a friend's place. After 2 months of sleeping on a single bed with a 4-year-old and being 8 months pregnant, I went back to him."

Women who divorce face the material consequences of poverty. They find it difficult, if not impossible, to find work that provides a wage sufficient to maintain a household. The majority of single-parent women live well below the poverty line. In contrast, most men improve their financial situation following divorce.

Women also face the social consequences of decreased status and the stigma of failure. Determined to make the marriage work at any cost, they fear that to not do so paints them as "failures" to themselves and to others. Some have already "failed" at marriage once and brought with them a child. Battering or chronic fear is the price that some are willing to pay to maintain the social facade of respectability and greater financial stability to which marriage entitles them. For those who grew up in a context of male violence, abuse and intimidation are all but normal. Social pressure also exists for women who did separate to go back to their husbands and "make it a family again":

"Even now, when I look back, I guess I was determined to make the marriage work, no matter what. And here again, I guess I felt had to prove it to my family that I wasn't a failure. I just wonder these days how much of that made me put up with what I did, because I put up with absolute hell."

"My first marriage failed and I was determined the second one wasn't going to fail, and I did love Ben very much, and I was prepared to put a lot of effort into it. I'm very stubborn. Once I've got my teeth in, it really takes a lot to let go."

"My father, his was verbal abuse, plus there were tantrums similar to my husband's, like slamming doors. We went to go away on a holiday. It was so traumatic with the screaming and yelling, packing the gear . . . and I've seen him kick the dog and belt my dog with the chain. I was so frightened of my father, the violence in him. So, in a way, I was prepared to put up with a little, with that, thinking it was normal with my husband, because I hadn't been shown any different."

"I did have friends. I don't class them as friends any more, and they'd visit Peter in jail, and they've been pushing and pushing and saying, 'It doesn't matter how Donny feels, I think you'd better go back when Peter gets out of jail and live with Peter and make it a family again, because Donny's only got a few more years with you, then he'll be off your hands, and what are you going to do with the rest of your life?'!"

The "loss of face" concept and an orientation toward the family rather than the individual may also inhibit women from Asian cultures from reporting violence out of concern that the family clan will lose respect and status. Instead, the partner's violence may remain hidden within the family and a harmonious public front presented to the world (Ho, 1990).

History of racism and consequent distrust of authorities constrains many minority women from seeking help to end the violence by reporting their own people to law officers or seeking help from social services (Ho, 1990). For these women, their own extended family network may offer the most protection, and it is the immigrant woman who is disconnected from her extended family who is at greatest risk, particularly if she is in a community that supports male dominance (Lau, 1986).

The difficulties for women in leaving violent husbands is not solely due to material or social factors. Many describe an intense attachment to their husband or ex-husband and relate many positive moments to the relationship, times during which the husband appears charming, loving, and a good husband or father:

"He can be a very loving and kind, good-hearted person. He was terrific with the kids. We went out. We had some really horrendous times in our family life but we had some really good ones, too, and they sort of, I suppose, in some ways, balanced out."

"I used to get panicky inside, and then I used to think, 'Well, I'll have to leave Ben and take the children with me,' and then he'd suddenly get out of that cycle and be the charming, good father, good husband, and the next minute, he'd be all crazy again."

"It was only at times; other times he was terrific and I really loved him. And I'd plead with him to come back, I'd get down on my knees, almost, and take the blame for everything, and it didn't take long. I'd believe it was my fault he drank, it was my fault he was how he was, you know?"

"John can be very good to you when he's, you know, when he's loving, he can be very good to you, he's a gentleman."

At its deepest level, however, the bond between the two is cemented upon the woman's perception of the man's vulnerability, her desire to care for him, and her perception of responsibility for his behavior. A woman's sympathy and concern are evoked by knowledge of her husband's difficult childhood, his lack of significant emotional connections to others, the assaults to his masculinity, such as his apparent lack of success in a male world, problems such as disability or unemployment, and by the perception of his "hurt":

"I've got a soft side for strays, animals, children, so that probably had a bit to do with it, too. If anybody's hurting, they can get around me very easily. So I've probably been vulnerable. That's why I could never kick John when he's down, could never kick him out the door and say, 'Bye-bye,' because you could see the hurt in him."

"I felt sorry for him, probably because his parents told him they didn't want to know him any more and they didn't care, and everybody had turned their back on him. But I've never forgiven him for what he'd done to Donny, but at the same time I felt sorry for him. I don't know, I just feel sorry for other people and their problems. You might just as well say that I'd help anybody out that's in trouble, you know."

"He's got nowhere to go . . . so he's out on the street. He can't work, because he's got nowhere to go. I said, 'Well, you can go to your mother's.' But he doesn't want to do that. He thinks that we're his life. If he goes, he said, 'I may as well be dead. I'll kill myself.' "

Despite the difficulties for women in leaving marriages, many marriages do come to an end. In some cases, the husband's battering of the wife or children reaches a point where the woman decides to leave. In others, the husband abandons the family to begin another relationship. In still other cases, the marriage reaches a crisis after revelations that force the woman to reconstruct her understanding of the relationship: The husband's well-kept secret history of sexual infidelity is revealed or, most devastatingly, children disclose that the father has been sexually assaulting them. At the point of this crisis and under the threat of the wife leaving, some couples seek therapy for the first time. In many other cases, however, women bring the marriage to an end.

This group of women, aged in their 30s and 40s, alone with their children following the breakup of their marriages, comprised the third major group of parents involved with CP services. Stresses for these women include coping with their children on their own, financial hardship, in some cases, the continuing conflict and negotiations inherent in separating from their husbands, and in others, the emotional and legal repercussions that flow from their child's disclosure of sexual assault. Single parenting is often a transient but still difficult phase. Although some women remain separated for a period of several years, others soon begin pairing off with new male partners.

Shortly after the separation or at the point where one of the children reaches adolescence or discloses sexual abuse, the children may become insolent, disobedient, and constantly testing of the limits set by the mother. For some mothers, these problems emerge for the first time following the separation. For others, they are part of a continuing escalation of the "contest of wills" previously described. Women who have held little authority with the children prior to the separation find it difficult to assert any authority afterward. Furthermore, mothers report that children who remain in contact with their fathers are often encouraged to disobey rather than to comply with their mothers' requests, as these mothers described:

> "When the two boys were little, I had to protect them from their father with his drinking and bashing them and abusing them, and I've sort of been mother and father to them, and my door is always open to them . . . but then when they come home, they hurt me so much, and the things I see them doing!"

> "The father's causing a lot of the problem. He virtually encourages them in a lot of things. I told Mark he couldn't go out at nighttime because he wanted to go out and stay out all the time. He would just ring up his father and say, 'Come and get me,' and his father would come and get him. And if I told them they couldn't do something, they would just ring him up."

Some women come to the attention of child protection authorities when neighbors witness them hitting or continually yelling at the children. Others present to a professional, saying that they cannot cope or are about to do their children harm. Some want financial relief, some want someone to talk to, and others simply want the problem child to be taken away. All feel they have "lost control," perhaps of their lives and certainly of their children. The sense of losing control shakes a deeply ingrained premise concerning parent–child relationships.

THE CONTROL OF CHILDREN

Regardless of family structure, age, gender, or marital status, with few exceptions, working-class parents maintain that parents must remain "in control" of children. Physical punishment is seen as a necessary aspect of managing children's behavior. The differential in size and strength between parents and children means that smacking is an effective way to assert such control, to state effectively, as one mother put it, "that you are not an adult, you are a child, and we are in control." Smacking was seen to do children good, as these women described:

> "I think a child does need a good smack now and again. No, I think a good smack never hurt any child. . . . A smack does them good. I've always believed that. There's nothing wrong with smacking a child. If you want that child under control, then that's the only way."

> "Because when I was a kid, and I mean when I was a kid it was tough. But what's wrong with being tough on a kid? It's the best way. . . . Yet kids today, they're allowed to get away with what they like. . . . Kids are just not doing what they're told, there's too many getting into trouble, into drugs and everything."

> "She [the CP Worker] says, 'Have you ever smacked your child?' I said, 'Yes, of course, I have. I've got three. All kids need a smack every now and then.' This 24-year-old girl said, 'You should never smack your children under any circumstances whatsoever.' I just thought that was a bit of crap. She doesn't know what she's talking about. . . . I think every child needs a smack when they're naughty, you know, when they do something they know is wrong, fighting and hitting another kid or something like that. I reckon that they should, you know, within reason. I reckon if I was too harsh, they wouldn't want to be with me, eh?"

Women frequently differentiate between "smacking" and "bashing." Smacking is defined as physical discipline called upon when the child "deserves it" and in order to return the child's behavior to acceptable standards. "Bashing," on the other hand, is less an attempt to change the child's behavior and more a way for the parent to discharge frustration by "taking it out on the children." Whereas smacking is said to be done with control and leaves no permanent physical damage, bashing can cause injuries and occurs when parents "lose control," as these mothers explained:

"I think a battered baby, as they call it, or used to call it, is completely different to giving a child a belting because he has done something wrong and you want to impress on him that that is not the way our family goes on."

"Some parents might call it slapping, but they're not actually slapping; they're actually bashing their kids. You know, you can actually hit a kid without bruising it, and then again, you can hit a kid and permanently do damage. So there's a natural difference to a smack, to child bashing. . . . If I get alcohol in me and smack the kids, to me, it feels like I'm bashing my kids because I've got that effect of alcohol in me and I've got no control. Everything just lets loose on me."

"*Child abuse* to me is obviously using cigarette burns and putting them in scalding water, brutally attacking them with some sort of instrument in the house, throwing their head against something that would hurt their head. But smacking them, in terms of smacking them with your hand, let's face it, when you're really angry and you're using your hand, you can only do it for so long before your arm gets very tired and you realize you've had enough. . . . If you're really that angry with the child and you really wanted to hurt the child, you wouldn't use your hand. You'd use something else. . . . "

Whether an incident is considered "smacking" or "bashing" depended upon the limits each parent draws in defining when smacking becomes bashing. The mother just quoted saw no problem with prolonged and severe spanking until "your arm gets very tired," so long as she used only her hand and no other implements. For other parents, belts or sticks are acceptable implements. Within some families, parents disagree with each other concerning what constitutes appropriate limits, most often mothers criticizing fathers for being too hard or, as one mother described it, "heavy-handed":

"My husband has always had a very heavy hand. He's never been light handed . . . and to him it's just like smacking. . . . When he goes to smack them, there's no control in his hand. . . . "

Parents also differ in their perceptions of the age at which smacking becomes an appropriate form of discipline. Smacking is sometimes used with infants much too young to comprehend the meaning of the parent's actions. The following mother saw nothing wrong with smacking her 8-month-old baby who, it later became evident, was allergic to his formula and cried constantly. Smacking a baby was acceptable so long as it was not down to the "hard skin":

"She said, 'Did you smack him?' and I said, 'Yes,' and she said, 'Where?' And I said, 'Through two nappies and a whole outfit.' She said, 'Do you realize what sort of impact that had on the child?' And I stood up with tears in my eyes and I said, 'You're not a mother. You wouldn't have any idea of what the frustration must be like, and I doubt whether that child would have even felt it. He knew he was being smacked, but definitely not to the hard skin.' "

Nor was she apparently aware of the possibility of brain damage resulting from shaking an infant:

"I never laid a hand on that child. I might have shaken him, I might have dumped him in the cot many a time through frustration, but I did not beat him. I did not ever slap him to the stage where he did not know what to do with himself."

In another case, a father, now serving a sentence for assault, routinely smacked his 9-month-old infant as "a warning not to cry through the night." When the child was teething, these "smacks" became increasingly severe, as the child's grandmother reported:

"She used to get smacked every night before she went to bed. That was a warning not to cry through the night. I was getting Sammy's tea ready, and she was griping a bit like she is now. She was teething, and he threatened to belt her. He took her into my bedroom, and I followed him in because I knew he would hit her. I pretended to get a tea towel out of the closet, and he punched her in the mouth. Her little mouth was all bleeding and that side of her face was all swollen and black, and there's marks under her little chin."

Parents from a minority culture often have further reasons for wanting to maintain strict discipline enforced through physical punishment. African American parents fear the lure of street crime and violence that is ever presently available to poor African American urban youth. Keeping their children in line and well behaved is seen to be a way of protecting them from the severe consequences of acting out behavior (Boyd-Franklin, 1989). Immigrant parents may also resort to physical punishment as a way of reasserting parental authority and controlling an adolescent who appears to be succumbing to the sexual dangers of Western culture when they associate with the opposite sex without parental supervision (Lau, 1986).

Despite parents' beliefs in the effectiveness of physical discipline, there is significant evidence that it does not achieve the aims parents desire. The use of severe physical discipline is associated with aggressive behavior in children and inconsistency in limit setting by parents. In two-parent situations, harsh or erratic treatment of a child by one parent is likely to result in the other parent subverting the first parent's authority and, therefore, in inconsistent limit setting (Henggeler & Borduin, 1990). In families where attention for desirable behavior is otherwise lacking, negative attention, including hitting, frequently reinforces the very behavior parents are trying to eliminate, escalating both the child's behavior and the parents' hitting. Children's behavior is often more than simply "willful defiance." Their activity and disobedience appears to increase in situations where parents are stressed or in conflict with each other, the mother is depressed and withdrawn, or sibling rivalry is intense. In each case, undesirable behavior exhibited by the child appears to activate the parent and focus attention on the child, away from more threatening areas. The parent's response to the child, although negative and physically painful, is nevertheless further reinforcement for the undesired behavior. Last, children who behave defiantly and aggressively are sometimes victims of sexual abuse (Sgroi, 1982). Physical discipline as a solution to their behavior is likely to further alienate them from the non-sexually abusive parent.

Parents who use physical force in disciplining describe receiving support for their views from sources within their social milieu. Neighboring families have similar views, and corporal punishment is still used in some schools. Some parents describe receiving support for the use of smacking from other authorities, lawyers, doctors, the police, psychologists, and even, one inferred, from a magistrate:

> "I've also spoken to our family lawyer about John stealing. . . . He said as a parent, I would do exactly the same [belt him]. And I said, 'Look, we've been up to the police station, and their idea was give the kid a boot in the bum,' and I said, 'Well, that's more or less what Peter did. He got a stick and hit him. He hit him with the feather duster, and the police said, 'Yes, that's what we would do.' . . . And when I told the Department they said, 'Oh, if you knew the number of policemen's children that we have to deal with, because that is the

attitude, you would be amazed.' . . . The police at the station told us, 'The kid's 9 years old. He deserves a boot in the bum for stealing.' "

"We took her to a doctor. . . . He had a look at her and even *he* turned around and said, 'If she was my child she'd end up with a few bruises.' Now he said that in front of the District Officer. Now why didn't that District Officer say something then? He just turned around and he laughed at what the doctor said. That if she was his child, 'she'd cop a few bruises herself' . . . and yet we're getting slammed down for actually doing it!"

One mother recalled how the family court counselor who assessed the family in preparation for the divorce settlement had explained to the children the necessity of parents' smacking:

"She had just said in her report that there was nothing wrong with smacking a child. She even told the four children that. She had 'em all lined up. She said, 'Do you realize that it is sometimes very necessary for Mummy or Daddy to smack you! Now that smacking can sometimes be across the face; they don't mean to be so hurtful, but you can make them so angry because you have not done what you've been told to do.' . . . The clinical psychologist put it into words: 'It is very necessary to smack your children; it is very necessary to teach them respect and to teach them discipline. There is a difference between smacking your child, hitting your child, bashing your child, and abusing your child.' "

Given the apparent social acceptance of corporal punishment, some parents said they were incredulous to discover that an authoritative government department had policies against hitting children. As one mother argued:

"I think they should have agreed with us that the child had done wrong and had to be punished in some manner that he would understand that if he did it again he would get hit again, but there was this idea that you don't hit children. I didn't know that that was one of their policies, that you don't hit children! . . . And you know that they say you can be charged for that?!"

The interpretation of what constitutes abuse, of when hitting becomes assault, is perceived as a debate that is far from settled:

"The Department don't believe in it at all. I was told the night they took the children that it was against the law to smack the children.

And they said that in court, too. The judge didn't know anything about it because I could tell by the way his eyes opened right up and he looked around and, you know, as if saying, 'Since when?' And then, half a grin comes on his face and he was looking all around like as if he was really enjoying the court case! So I thought at least I wasn't the only one who didn't know!"

"He [the lawyer] said, 'Rubbish! Rubbish! In 16 years they'll all be up here for murder,' he said. 'You just can't let kids get away with things.' And one of the officers from the Department said, 'If you let them get away with things, it will all be out of their system by the time they're 16.'"

The notion of control is not simply an idea that lives independently in the minds of individual parents. It is kept alive by the social sanctions that are applied when parents do not appear to be in control. Children who are rude, argumentative, disobedient, aggressive, who lie, steal, and show little respect for authority or the property of others are identified by relatives, neighbors and school authorities as "problem children." Relatives respond by criticizing the parents' management of the child, both to the parents and to other members of the extended family. Relatives offer advice or deal with the child directly, further adding to the child's sense of confusion and the parents' feeling of inadequacy. Neighbors respond by not permitting their children to play with the problem child, and by withdrawing socially from the child's parents. Schools respond by regularly reporting to the mother on the child's intolerable behavior, and, at some point, referring the family to counseling for "their problem" or threatening to suspend the child if the parents do not "do something." One mother described the isolation and sense of stigma she experienced when her son's behavior was out of control:

"Well the first thing is your kids aren't behaving themselves very well, so other parents tell their kids not to play with them. Other mothers don't come to you and say, 'Oh, Olivia, you're having trouble. Is there anything I can do to help?' The first thing people do is run. 'Oh, they're having a problem, we don't want to know about it!' ... It makes the problem 10 times worse. Your kids are acting ratty and you've got nobody to even go and sort of have coffee with, no time out or anything like that. You're stuck in a totally isolated situation to a point where, you know, you are going up to the school and nobody will even sort of say hello to you. Stigma's not the word for it! Yeah, a gigantic stigma! People don't want to have contact with you because if you *do* make the mistake of trying, *trying* to be friendly, people will openly snub you. If you say, 'Hi,' they say, 'I've got to go now,' and they just about leave skid marks taking off."

Parents fear that uncontrollable children will become uncontrollable adolescents who will short circuit their life chances as adults through the consequences of teenage pregnancy, premature termination of education or incarceration, situations often known only too well by the parents. For the working-class father, who makes meaning of his work as a sacrifice for his children's future life chances, and for the working-class mother, whose only sense of control is often to be found in the parental realm, an uncontrollable child is evidence of their failure.

In overviewing their life contexts, it becomes apparent that many of the women who become clients of child protection authorities live lives that are overshadowed at each stage by violence. Their families might be termed, as Luepnitz (1988) has coined it, patriarchal, yet father-absent. Although they are not a representative sample of family life in the Western world, these families do represent one end of the continuum of normal family life in a patriarchal context, a context in which fathers are constructed by the demands of "masculinity" and the workplace and, although emotionally dependent on their wives, are often left on the periphery of the intense relationship between women and children, and a context in which women, unprepared for self-sufficiency and overburdened with domestic labor and child care, are expected to be "in control" of children to whom they turn for emotional support. The ideology of coercion and control, whether or not ever reaching the point of overt violence, permeates the fabric of family life. But so does the discourse of femininity and the family that constructs women as responsible for providing the care and maintenance of the family unit, even if at their own expense.

As therapists, we are still left with the following question: Why is it that children are abused within some working-class families, while in others they are not? To answer these questions, we must address the specific differences between families that account for why abuse becomes an option in a particular family at a particular time. This takes us to the genealogy of relationships, discussed in the following chapter.

The Genealogy
of Relationships

IN the previous chapter, I described the discourse of the family and how
it impacts upon the working class, creating particular patterns of relationships between men and women, parents and children. I also illustrated
how these patterns of behavior are cemented into cultural notions of
femininity and masculinity, and thus deeply embedded into the individual's sense of identity and sense of adequacy as a person. In addition to a
lens that illuminates the experience of life in a working-class context, we
also need a lens that positions individuals as active subjects in an
interactional context and that can account for incongruity and conflict
within the person. The lens we use is the genealogical method.

Consider the following: Erick is a 30-year-old male, who, after
completing high school, became employed as a repair man doing what he
described as "dirty hands" work. He has been married for 8 years to his
wife, Claire, and they have one daughter, age 7. Before they married, Erick
and Claire traveled briefly and in the course of their travels became
involved in political activities in a Third World country. This experience
opened their eyes to another way of seeing the world and had bonded
them closely. Both Erick and Claire developed an alternative ideal to the
patriarchal husband–wife relationships they had seen in their own families
of origin. Erick henceforth professed to want a marriage of equality. He
perceived his wife as intelligent and talented, and her success and
advancement in the world became as important to him as his own. He
felt this to such a degree, he said, that if her success meant leaving him
behind, "she should do it." He would "push her to do it."

Years later, however, Claire did, in a sense, begin to leave Erick
behind. Although Erick also advanced and was promoted to foreman,
Claire sought further training and landed a new job in which she was

rapidly promoted. Her work began to entail close association with white collar professional men whom Erick considered to have "clean" jobs. He noticed that Claire began to dress better, more attractively, to go to work. In bed, she seemed to "change," she was different. While claiming to be proud of her success, Erick began to obsess about her going to work each day, and he developed what appeared to be a delusion that she was having an affair with her boss. He became moody and short-tempered with Claire and their daughter. One day, in a fury at her "betrayal," he hit her as she was preparing to leave for work. When their daughter cried and protested, Erick accused her of covering up for her mother's activities. Erick slapped her across the face and sent her sprawling to the floor.

Under physical threat from Erick, and under pressure from his claim of betrayal, in the end, Claire decided to quit her job. Erick said he was willing to forgive her for the "affair," but Claire would not lower herself to admit an infidelity that she had not committed. Feeling trapped and frightened, she sought therapy.

In therapy, it became clear that Erick's delusion of the "affair" was his solution to what was for him an otherwise irresolvable conflict. On the one hand, his commitment and attachment to the ideal of equality in marriage was profound. He reasserted with passion his commitment to Claire's success in life, even if it meant that she left him behind. On the other hand, as a working-class man, he held the deeply ingrained premise that individual worth is based upon individual ability and that his own lack of success in the world resulted from his lack of ability. When asked how he thought Claire would see him if she were to become even more successful and important at her job, he said that he believed she would look at him as an inferior sort of person, and she would become more attracted to "clever men" working in "clean" jobs.

Had Erick led a more ordinary life, never traveled, never embraced new values, he would not have found himself in such conflict. He would simply have asserted his right as a male and husband to stop his wife from working at a job that positioned her socially at a higher level than himself. Erick, however, could not face doing something so antithetical to his belief in the equality. So instead, in order to end his turmoil, Erick became fixated on the idea that Claire had betrayed him by having an extramarital affair. He felt entitled to assert himself against this type of betrayal because it was not incongruent with his ideal of equality. This allowed him to redress what he experienced as the powerlessness and unfairness of his position. Although he felt regret and remorse at having "lost control" and hurt his wife and daughter, he thought it was only right and proper that Claire quit her job in order to end the "affair" with her boss.

Erick was the site of conflicting discourses about masculinity and gender relationships. His dependency and the intensity of his attachment to Claire generated intense feelings of powerlessness when he felt himself to be in a context in which his "success" could be measured and judged. These feelings of powerlessness became a crucial stimulus to action.

Possibly more than any other context, relationships within the family are capable of generating extreme feelings of powerlessness. The most intense of these feelings arise from within those situations in which someone feels excluded, rejected, or abandoned by other important family members. Feelings of powerlessness also arise when the person feels incapable or ambivalent about carrying out the actions dictated by the requirements of a discourse in which they are immersed. A mother who expects to feel powerful in relation to a child because "it is the duty of parents to control children," will feel powerless and inadequate in the face of evidence that she is not in control. A man who expects to feel powerful in his family because "a man should be respected as head of the family," will feel threatened and powerless in the face of apparent disrespect from his wife or children. On the other hand, individuals can also feel powerless because they cooperate with the dictates of a discourse—a woman marries, albeit to a man she doesn't love; a man works daily at hard and humiliating work—and in the process subjugate other needs, desires, and wants.

Social factors may contribute to and compound feelings of powerlessness. Non-English-speaking immigrant parents may feel a great loss of control as their maturing and socially adept children become increasingly able to "hoodwink" them. Couple relationships may deteriorate as the male partner experiences ongoing humiliation and powerlessness in the face of extended unemployment.

In the face of intense feelings of powerlessness, individuals are very likely to resist, and this resistance will often take the form of actions intended to make them feel powerful. This is not to say that these individuals, *in fact*, lack actual material power, despite their feelings of powerlessness. Nor is it to say that what an individual does to resist, in fact, makes him or her more powerful. An individual acts from within the experience of power or powerlessness rather than from within an outsider's "objective" assessment of the extent of that person's power.

In our experience, the abuse of a child is intimately connected to shifts in family alliances in which one person perceives him- or herself as powerless in the face of being excluded, rejected, or neglected. The resulting, often unspoken conflict both triggers the person who becomes abusive and initiates or escalates relationship struggles within the family as individuals attempt to rectify their powerlessness or retaliate against perceived unfairness. Family members' responses to experiencing or witnessing abuse and their resultant experience of powerlessness feed back into the interaction, creating further relationship shifts and either escalating or in some way resolving the initial relationship struggles. The shift in relationships, the ensuing conflict, and family members' responses to the abuse interact recursively. It is this focus on the history of relationship struggles that lies at the heart of a genealogical method.[1]

THE GENEALOGICAL METHOD

Within each particular family, there is a discourse that functions as "the truth." Discourses do not arise out of a vacuum but are intimately connected to social discourses concerning the family, heterosexuality, masculinity, and femininity. The discourse defines what it is possible to say, what it is possible to think, and how events are to be interpreted. The dominant definition of the "problem" emerges from within this discourse. This definition along with the related explanations for the problem, constitute what I will call the "dominant account."

Instead of "truth," the genealogical method is concerned with the function of interpretation in serving the interests of maintaining the dominant views or discourses. It seeks to uncover the play of wills in the forms of subjugation and domination within a network of relationships in constant tension and activity. Although the genealogical method is about understanding the operation of power, it does not construct actors as occupying fixed roles of "power" and "victim" but perceives all actors as constantly engaged in tactics, strategies, and maneuvers (Dreyfus & Rabinow, 1986; Foucault, 1980, 1984).[2]

The problem is tracked back to the time of conflict when the experience or views of certain individuals in the family became subjugated or lost. It is this "painstaking rediscovery of the struggle, together with the rude memory of their conflict" (Foucault, 1980, p. 83) that begins the process of exploring and making space for those subjugated voices. In bringing to the fore this conflict and holding it at center stage, thus speaking what before was unspeakable, tolerating what before was intolerable, some new resolution that is less authoritarian, less rigid, and less abusive can be voiced.

In unraveling the history of conflicts, and in an understanding of subjectivity created through discourses, it becomes apparent that "problems" frequently represent some form of resistance against the dominant discourse. The problem a child's behavior presents to his or her parents

---

[1] This is a method of sociological analysis associated with Michel Foucault (1980, 1984) and modified by us for its use in a clinical context.

[2] This is not to say that there is not such a thing as domination, but that even within situations of domination, the dominated one actively resists the dominator.

and "the problem" of a parent's abusive behavior toward the child may both be forms of resistance taken up against the current dominant discourse. Although one group or person may appear to "succeed" by suppressing certain views and maintaining the dominant account, this position of power generates its own resistance. When the context is one in which opposition cannot be safely expressed, resistance is disguised and, although appearing foreign and disconnected, nevertheless works at eroding the dominant source of power.

Subjugation and resistance are thus multifold across relationships and within individuals. Here, the landscape can be confusing for the therapist. The man who rules his family autocratically generates resistance from other family members. At some stage, he has the tables turned on him as his wife and children turn against him, and he becomes alienated from those he is most afraid to lose. He cannot speak of these fears or admit his need for connection in the face of that part of himself that must, at all costs, be seen as masculine. But in repressing this part of himself, it reemerges, resisting its own subjugation, taking hold with a symptom such as the compulsion to sexually assault, which he experiences as beyond his control.

From the point of view of those benefiting the most from the dominant account (e.g., the autocratic father) the reemergence of suppressed conflict is, at least, threatening to the stability, the security, and the power of their position. From the perspective of those benefiting least (e.g., the wife and children of the autocratic father), the reemergence of the conflict may be experienced as a great relief—their experience, which has been denied and invalidated, has finally been given voice. This relief, however, is tinged with the fear and anxiety associated with possible consequences. Facing and reworking the conflict is only undertaken by family members at a particular point in time, because the consequence of not doing so are experienced as more threatening.

Dominant accounts draw from and mirror prevailing values and beliefs within the family and cultural context. Hidden accounts, on the other hand, represent those voices both within an individual and within families that are silenced. Within families, subjugation occurs in the case of young children who have never had the authority or understanding to speak. Youths and adults may participate more actively in their own subjugation, simply because they are silenced in the face of threats and intimidation from other family members.

Within each individual, internal voices are inevitably silenced, because each person is simultaneously defined by different and often competing discourses. An "individual" is not a unified subject but is comprised of multiple, competing, and often contradictory wants, needs, and desires. These wants, needs, and desires are constructed through different social discourses, discourses that may be in conflict with each other. Subjectivity is thus constituted by contradictory identities; that is, subjectivity is split and multiple. An individual's choice at a particular time to bring forward one aspect of him- or herself—that is, one identity—and thus to privilege it over other competing wants/needs/desires or to enact a "compromise" between contradictory desires is what at any one given moment gives the appearance of unity.

Power, however, generates resistance. The privileging of one aspect of self over other important aspects in some ways generates resistance and attempts to sabotage the dominant view. At any one time, with the change in the relational context or through greater exposure to a different discourse, an individual may reconstruct him- or herself differently by bringing forward background wants, needs, or desires. There are differences between individuals and between families in the degree of disunity. This reflects the degree to which one part or person in the conflict has been suppressed in the interests of the dominant view.

In therapy, the stability of the dominant account can be undermined by teasing apart and reconstructing the history of dominant accounts—the history of important struggles—using the genealogical method. This is an interactional process between therapist and family members in which successive layers of interpretation or meaning are uncovered by tracking events and their meanings over time. In unraveling the genealogy of relationships, we are interested in four levels of description:

Level 1. The initial account of the problem and family relationships, and the subsequent accounts as therapy progresses.

Level 2. Temporal events and the meaning attributed to these events by different parties.

Level 3. The meaning the events have since taken on via background discourses that crucially determine how individuals understand themselves (i.e., the creation of subjectivity).

Level 4. The needs, desires, and wants of individuals and how these are formed by or in conflict with discourses and individual histories.

THE CONSTRUCTION OF SUBJECTIVITY

One of the primary ways discourses construct subjectivity is through a network of premises that are actively incorporated by the individual. These premises are taken up in emotionally powerful relationship contexts and are thus not easily altered or changed. In our use of the term, a premise is a basic assumption, not usually consciously articulated, from which inferences are drawn about the workings of the world. Beliefs and explanations, on the other hand, are conscious constructions, usually presented as rational, that may either reflect or conflict with the underlying network of premises. Discourses and the resulting premises contribute to the arousal of affective states. For example, if, as is consistent within the discourse of masculinity, a man operates by the premise that he should be treated like a king in his own home, he will feel the affective states of anger, hurt, and rejection when he is not treated in this way. If he also happens to consciously believe in the equality of women, his subjectivity will be split. This is one way in which discourses construct subjectivity. Premises can also conflict with needs, desires, and wants, and result in their repression. For example, a man who operates by the premise that it is not acceptable for men to show vulnerability will repress feelings of sadness when he perceives himself as rejected. Needs, wants, and desires, themselves, however, are not biological or natural givens. Their particular construction and shape is also mediated through interaction and discourses, and past and current family relationships.

The relationship of any two premises, or between a premise and a belief, may be complementary; that is, although different, they do not challenge or invalidate the other. Alternatively, premises and beliefs may be in opposition or mutually exclusive to each other, thus producing inconsistency in behavior and the experience of internal conflict. For example, as described in the case of Erick and Claire, a man may, on the one hand, believe that he and his wife are equals. He firmly asserts that his wife should have the same options and opportunities as he, himself, has. Yet, when his wife begins to become more successful than he is, he experiences a faltering in his sense of masculinity, fears losing her, and actively seeks to constrain her from her work. The premise underlying his behavior (and possibly not consciously available to him), is that a man must occupy a socially superior position to his wife or risk being rejected by her in favor of more attractive (i.e., socially superior) men.

The relationship between the network of premises and beliefs held by one person and others within a family is more complex. Some premises and beliefs may be *shared*. For example, all family members may operate on the premise that it is dangerous to trust outsiders. Other premises and beliefs may be complementary. A couple, for example, may hold different but complementary premises regarding emotional closeness. She may operate from the premise that if she gets close, she will be abandoned, and he, from the premise that if he gets close, he will be suffocated. They adopt a distant relationship that threatens neither of them. In other instances, contradictory premises result in conflict. She may interpret his refusal to talk as abandonment, while he experiences intense communication as suffocating. Thus, he distances, and she feels abandoned and rejected. They argue over the perceived faults of the other. In all of these situations, both parties maintain *other* premises and beliefs that may be shared, complementary, or conflictual.

Networks of premises tend to maintain a sense of coherence across time and through most relationship contexts. The significance of particular beliefs, however, can change over time. New beliefs may be adopted or earlier beliefs withdrawn as individuals are exposed to new situations in which different discourses circulate. However, those aspects of identity and the corresponding network of premises concerned with gender, sexuality, and parent–child relationships are not easily changed. This is because, first, they are produced within powerful emotional contexts, and second, because they reflect elements of discourse so commonplace that they are accepted as everyday "truths," and may thus be invisible even to the therapist.

A genealogical understanding of relationships and the construction of subjectivity is best illustrated through the case example that follows.

CASE EXAMPLE: THE NICOLOPOULOS FAMILY

George and Fatima Nicolopoulos sought therapy after their 16-year-old daughter, Gloria, disclosed to Fatima that George had recently attempted to touch her genitals when he had driven her home from her ballet lessons. Fatima confronted her husband, who admitted the allegations and moved out of the home at Fatima's request. George said he was ashamed of his behavior and could give no explanation for it. Fatima then initiated therapy, hoping to get help for her husband so that he could return home.

The couple had three other children, a daughter 18, who had left home the previous year, and two sons aged 14 and 12. George had been employed as a machinery repairman for the last 20 years, and Fatima worked as a retail sales clerk. George's father was of Greek descent and his mother was Anglo-Australian. Fatima was of Lebanese descent.

The Story of the Abuse

Fatima described her husband as controlling, intimidating, and verbally abusive. She resented his tight hold over the family finances and disagreed with his extreme control over the children's social activities. Fearing that his daughters would be vulnerable to sexual exploitation, he had prevented them from engaging in any social activities where boys would be present. The eldest daughter had rebelled and left home the previous year. Fatima said she believed that the children "should have a chance to know what life is about," since she, herself, had "got married young and didn't know anything." She was nevertheless afraid to openly disagree with George.

George appeared surprised that Fatima described him as so controlling. From his perspective, the decisions they made were generally "50–50. She knows it's by mutual agreement." Fatima rarely disagreed with or challenged his views directly, and he perceived her submission as agreement. He said that it was the man's responsibility to provide financial support for the family, and he resented the fact that Fatima spent money without telling him. Feeling unappreciated and unwanted by both his wife and children, whom he perceived as banding together against him, he said he was "regarded as the bread supply."

When interviewed separately, Gloria, age 16, and her 12- and 14-year-old brothers described feeling afraid of their father's verbal intimidation and violent outbursts. They said their relationship to their father was "different" than other father–adolescent relationships, in that their father never spoke to them. Angry that their eldest sister had left home after arguments with their father, they felt trapped and hopeless.

Both the sons and the daughter resented that all of the household work fell on the shoulders of their mother, despite the fact that both parents had paid employment. Their father also expected them to wait on him at home. He seemed to control all the important decisions about them and their mother. On the rare occasions when the one of the sons had stood up to him, his father had beaten him.

We explored the onset of the struggle over autonomy and control, and tracked this back to the couple's courtship. Fatima described herself as growing up in a Lebanese family with a patriarchal father, whom she experienced as powerful and domineering. Both she, her siblings, and her mother feared him and accepted his rule. As an adolescent, she complied with her father's demand that she not date. George was a friend of her brother's with whom she began a secret relationship. After only a few episodes of unprotected intercourse, Fatima discovered she was pregnant. George wanted to marry her. Her father, however, was furious with Fatima for her secretiveness and betrayal, and forbade the marriage. He also rejected George because his family was not Lebanese, and because he believed that George's mother "lacked morals" (i.e., she was known to drink at a local pub). It was only when Fatima's brothers ganged up in a wall of silence against their father that he reconsidered the situation. Faced with the choice of Fatima marrying George or giving birth to a baby out of wedlock, Fatima's father relented. In the end, he consented to the wedding on the condition that George agree that Fatima and any child of the marriage would have no contact with George's parents or siblings. All children were also be raised within Fatima's family's church.

After the marriage, Fatima's parents continued to have significant influence over her. In an attempt to gain Fatima's respect and win her away from her family, George sought to be like Fatima's father, and he became increasingly controlling and intimidating.

George visited his parents alone over the next 18 years but grieved quietly that his children had never met their grandparents, aunts, or uncles. When George brought home his younger brother, Fatima refused to have him in the house. In the argument that ensued, George hit Fatima. She left the house and returned 1 week later. George never again broached the subject of his parents until this therapy, several years later. He never hit her again, but she remained fearful of him thereafter.

George described himself as feeling more important in the family when the children were younger. Although he was hard on the children, he believed that Fatima expected him to be that way and that he was doing his job as a father. As the children grew, however, and became more challenging of his decisions, he felt his authority slipping and his position as increasingly on the emotional periphery of the family. When their eldest daughter left home after arguing with him, he experienced Fatima as angry and withdrawing from him. His resentment and anger increased. Four months prior to commencing therapy, he became preoccupied with an idea—an idea that he later enacted and for which he appeared unable to account either to himself or to his wife and children. He stopped the car when he was driving his daughter home and sexually assaulted her. He became the very person he feared would violate his daughter's sexuality.

Background Discourses

We can see in this story the influence and expression of a number of background discourses. Both parents operated from the premise that it is natural for men to be dominant in relationships. They believed that a man has the responsibility to control and protect his daughters from sexual exploitation. Protection is seen as necessary, because it is believed that every man will attempt to sexually exploit women and that "good" women (unlike George's own mother) must not be seen as sexual outside of marriage. The control over Fatima's outings by her father, and, a generation later, her husband's adoption of similar practices in relation to his wife and children, was thus expected on one level by both George and Fatima. On the other hand, Fatima had the consistent belief that her children should have a chance to know what life is about. This was the chance she herself had not known, but it was one to which she (perhaps through the influence of feminist discourses within the community) believed she had been entitled. George's own subjectivity was revealed as split between "good" and "bad" when he became the very abuser from whom he had believed he was protecting his daughter.

In unraveling the genealogy of relationships in this case and the social discourses that underpin it (see Figure 5.1), we can begin with Fatima's experience of powerlessness, vis-à-vis her father and husband. Fatima's father (and later, her husband) believed in his right as a male to control his daughter's behavior in the name of "protection." Her father's control prevented her from exploring relationship possibilities, subjugating her desire, need, and right to have a partner of her own choosing. Fatima had always assumed she would marry but said she never had the chance to know whether George was the right man. Whereas on the one hand she felt trapped into marrying George, becoming pregnant could simultaneously be seen as a form of resistance to her father's power. The enforced marriage on one level robbed her of her freedom, whereas on another level, it simultaneously freed her from her father, whom she viewed as more patriarchal than George.

George's perception of Fatima's ambivalence about the relationship left him feeling insecure. Her submission to her father's demand that George relinquish his family meant that George had to subjugate his desire, need, and right to have both a wife and connection with his own family and siblings, and his own religious and ethnic heritage. His experience of this, however, was hidden because, on the face of it, George complied with Fatima's father.

Why did Fatima, some 18 years later, still insist upon George keeping his promise not to allow their children to see his parents? On the one hand, Fatima still submitted to her father's wishes. On the other hand, submitting to this particular demand of her father's gave her leverage in relation to her husband. As much as he dominated her, she could resist his dominance, even if only in this small but crucial area. Thus, there was a space in which she could experience some autonomy.

Over time, Fatima and the children responded to George's increasing control of their independent expressions of activities by drawing together and excluding him, which could be seen as a form of resistance. George had sacrificed his family of origin for his wife and children and now found himself rejected by them. The enforced separation between his children and his parents felt increasingly more intolerable. This account, however, remained hidden. Dealing with his feelings of rejection and anger in a masculine and instrumental manner, he ran his family like a business, keeping himself emotionally distant and apparently "invulnerable." The consequence of denying these apparently unacceptable feelings was their inevitable reemergence, this time in the form of sexual abuse. The sexual abuse of his daughter was simultaneously an expression of anger toward his wife and children, retaliation for what he experienced as his own

BACKGROUND
DISCOURSES   CONFLICTS

1. Whether Fatima's father should be controlling his daughter's relationships outside
   the family.

Patriarchal right of
father to control
daughter's sexuality.

| Father's surveillance of couple. | ⟷ | Fatima's compliance. | ⟷ | Her desire, need, and right to have a husband of own choosing. |

Resistance: Has secret relationship—gets pregnant.

2. Whether couple should be allowed to marry.

Women should
marry upward in
social class.
Sexualized
women are
devalued.

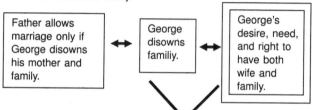

| Father allows marriage only if George disowns his mother and family. | ⟷ | George disowns familiy. | ⟷ | George's desire, need, and right to have both wife and family. |

Resistance: George competes with father for dominance.

3. Whether George should be able to control activities and expressions of Fatima
   and the children.

Father as head of
household.
Parents have right
and duty to
control children.
Marriage is equal
partnership, 50–50.

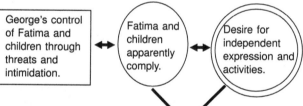

| George's control of Fatima and children through threats and intimidation. | ⟷ | Fatima and children apparently comply. | ⟷ | Desire for independent expression and activities. |

Resistance: Fatima withdraws and bands together with children.

4. Whether George should be excluded from family relationships.

It is natural for
women to be closer
to their children.
Men don't get upset,
express sadness or
loss. Men are
responsible for
providing financial
support.

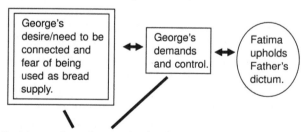

| George's desire/need to be connected and fear of being used as bread supply. | ⟷ | George's demands and control. | ⟷ | Fatima upholds Father's dictum. |

Resistance: Sexually assaults daughter.

FIGURE 5.1. Genealogy of relationships: The Nicolopoulos family.

victimization, as well as a reflection of his desire to be more intimate and involved with his family.

The operation of power creates its own resistance, in this case, an unexpected pregnancy resulting from a rebellious and "illicit" act against Fatima's father, and the sexual abuse of a daughter by her father who was expressing his rage against the control his wife and her father had over him. For George, the experience of powerlessness led him to assert and reassert his dominance, thus expressing the dominant discourse of masculinity. Fatima, on the one hand, powerless in the face of her husband's controlling and dominating behavior, passively resisted by excluding and rejecting him, rendering him powerless in return. Constructed by discourses concerning femininity and mothering, Fatima responded to her husband's control by becoming closer to their children.

CONCLUSION

This chapter has presented a genealogical approach to understanding the evolution of abuse within families. Like any other account of problems, a genealogical account is a *construction* by the therapist using information that is provided from family members' accounts in response to the therapist's questions. From our viewpoint, it is a preferred way of understanding abuse within families, because it takes account of the influence of background discourses and the interactional nature of family life. It avoids the pathologizing of individual family members, while nevertheless making sense of abuse as an individual's choice and responsibility within a conflictual relationship field. Importantly, a genealogical approach seeks and allows for each person's account of relationships and, as will be elaborated in Chapter 9, it can become a guide to how therapists can approach obtaining the story of abuse from family members and effect a change in underlying network premises held by family members.

In Part II of this book, I turn my attention from understanding the interconnection of child abuse, working-class life, and the particular genealogy of family relationships to the more pragmatic issue of setting the stage for successful therapy by earning the parents' trust, working with CP Workers, and eliciting and maintaining parents' motivation. This will be followed by a further explanation of aspects of a relationship-centered approach—rewriting the story of abuse and creating a relationship discourse.

PART TWO

THE THERAPIST
AS POWER BROKER

Initial Meetings:
Earning the Parents' Trust

RETURN for the moment to the story of Anna Ryan, whose difficult encounter with therapy and, before that, the Department, was described in Chapters 2 and 3. Anna was notified to the Department and ordered by the Courts to therapy. She resisted the therapist so successfully that despite the Court Order, the therapist "gave up" and suggested they stop meeting. It was at that point—the point where Anna believed she had some choice—that Anna chose to continue with the therapist, and therapy really began.

Anna's story taught us something about therapy with child-at-risk cases, something so simple and yet so profound that it changed how we approached all cases referred from the CP Department. It taught us, first, that the most important step the therapist must take is that of earning the parents' trust. Second, trust cannot be earned unless and until the therapist establishes a context in which the parents have some element of choice.

There are a number of important ways in which therapists can earn parents' trust and establish a structure for later work. In what follows, I discuss strategies for laying the groundwork for therapy by paying particular attention to first contacts, explaining the context of therapy and connecting with family members in a "meeting" prior to any "therapy." Criteria for the sharing of information between therapists and other professionals are proposed, and suggestions are made for how these criteria are to be clearly and honestly conveyed to clients. Finally, I describe how therapy must begin with framing parents' intentions positively and by offering assistance with problems as defined by parents, not by the therapist.

INITIAL MEETINGS:
LAYING THE GROUNDWORK

The first step in accepting a referral for therapy from the Department is to organize a meeting with the parents to discuss "whether we are the right people" for them. This initial meeting is an effective way to convey to parents that they have a real choice in deciding to work with the therapist, and it maximizes the possibility of the parents engaging in therapy.

Not all referrals from the Department involve coerced or reluctant referrals. Because however, it may be difficult to ascertain the degree to which the parents experience therapy as voluntary until the therapist has met with them and heard their story, we take a similar initial approach to therapy with all clients referred from the Department.

First Contacts

To begin on the right footing, it is important to have personal contact directly with parents and avoid intake procedures in which the parent enters into telephone discussions or assessment interviews with other workers prior to seeing the therapist. Personal contact conveys a sense of attention and concern while allowing the therapist the opportunity to perceive the situation afresh and to begin to create a "frame" from which the problem can be viewed. The person who is to act as the therapist, therefore, makes the first contact with the family. Usually, this involves returning a telephone call or following up on a referral from the Department. During this telephone call to one of the parents, the parents are invited to meet with the therapist prior to beginning therapy in order to decide "if we are the right people for you."

Prior to the initial meeting, it is only necessary to obtain a brief account from the referral source, which includes the genogram and a brief account of the problem. This allows the therapist to enter the pretherapy meeting unencumbered by preconceived ideas and also free to honestly disclose what information has been received without appearing aligned with the referral source.[1]

---

[1]In the early days of the project, we experimented with inviting the CP Workers to the initial meeting, believing that this would allow the CP Worker to directly define the problem and allow us to be perceived by the parents as separate from the Department. We abandoned this approach, however, after it became clear that both the parents and the CP Workers did not speak as openly during these meetings, and that the parents, in many cases, continued to see us an extension of the CP Worker.

Although it is important to ultimately obtain the perspectives of each family member, it is not always useful to bring the whole family together for the first meeting. In cases of sexual assault, in particular, it is appropriate to see family members in separate subsystems. In other situations, parents themselves are reluctant to include all members. Work commitments may make it difficult for the parent to attend, or parents may be reluctant to initially include all of their children. When parents raise these issues, they can be encouraged to bring whomever they wish to the initial meeting. The meeting can then be used to discuss the parents' concerns. Since it is a "meeting" rather than "therapy," seeing only one parent does not imply that therapy itself is possible without the other family members.

Explaining the Context of Therapy

In beginning the initial meeting, two tasks must be accomplished: (1) family members must be clearly informed about the context of therapy, and (2) the therapist must connect with each person present. Although, in practice, these two tasks are often intertwined, here we will consider each in turn, beginning with explaining the context of therapy.

Although it is often the practice of family therapists to work in teams, it is best to limit the initial meeting to one therapist and one colleague, both of whom sit in the interview room during the initial introductions and explanations. The purpose of the initial meeting is then explained in a manner that makes no presumptions that this meeting constitutes the beginning of therapy. Using "plain English," the therapist introduces him- or herself and the agency, clearly and honestly explaining any peculiarities about the room (e.g., one-way screens or video equipment) or the way of working (e.g., with one therapist behind the screen). At the end of these explanations, the parents may be asked if they would like to go ahead with this meeting. At various points throughout this interview, it is important that parents are offered choices, starting with the choice of whether to continue with this pretherapy meeting and ending with the choice about whether to make a further appointment. Figure 6.1 provides an edited and condensed version of a therapist explaining the context of therapy during the initial meeting.

It is important that parents be genuinely and noncoercively asked for their consent for such activities as videotaping or the second therapist moving to sit behind a one-way screen. It is easier not to use the videotape camera during this initial meeting, when connecting with family members remains the therapist's highest concern.

"What we would like to do is explain to you how we work, and talk with you about what you are wanting before we decide to go ahead. This place is called the Couple and Family Center. Some people think that we are an extension of the Department, but in fact are not. We are quite separate.

"Our job is to help families who have problems with their children. We also help families who have problems dealing with the Welfare. A lot of families have bad experiences dealing with professionals, and we would like to try to make that better. It can often be very confusing for families when they have many different professionals involved.

"What we would like to do today is to get to know you, have you get to know us, and hear your story about what has happened to you. At the end of our meeting today, you can decide whether you think this is the right place, and whether we are the right people to help you with the difficulties you have been having, so that you have a choice about whether you want to work with us."

FIGURE 6.1. An actual example of a therapist explaining the context of therapy.

Connecting with Family Members

When introducing themselves and explaining the context of therapy, therapists must find ways of conveying respect and connecting with each family member. Small but significant steps in this process include greeting and interacting with family members in a warm, interested manner, beginning the interview at the scheduled time, and not keeping the family waiting. After explaining the context of therapy, the therapist spends a few minutes asking each person about his or her work, school, or interests. This develops a connection with each person as an individual and often decreases anxiety. Importantly, it often helps the therapist relax and decrease his or her own anxiety. During these introductions, the conversation is kept focused on nonproblem areas before making a clear shift to the family's story.

Efforts to build rapport are sometimes misinterpreted by parents who have been coerced into attending therapy or have had previous negative experiences with therapists or other professionals. It is essential to actively avoid and defuse potential escalations by "leaning into" parents' anger, anticipating their reactions, responding with empathy, inquiring about their distress, taking a one-down position, and maintaining a quiet tone, eye contact, and an open body posture. Any therapist behavior that can be construed even slightly by the parents as blaming, criticizing, accusing, or disagreeing undermines the process of connecting.

In the following example, although the difficulties encountered are uncommon in that the mother's defensiveness was extreme, the transcript provides a useful example of building rapport in difficult circumstances.

This transcript was the first meeting with Anita Grey and her 13-year-old daughter, Sarah.[2]

THERAPIST: What I'd like to do before we get started is get to know you a little bit. It often helps us to==

ANITA: ==(*and groaning*) Oh, *here* we go again! Do you people not keep records? Wouldn't it be easier to just read the records instead of wasting time going through the whole history. Seriously, I don't mean to be facetious; it just seems a waste of time to go through the whole family's history time after time. Apart from that, it's quite traumatic for me to go through this time and time again.

THERAPIST: (*softly*) I wasn't referring to your history. I was actually referring to just getting to know you as a person==

ANITA: ==Fair enough! (*responding sarcastically and clapping her hands together*) You won't find much in me!

THERAPIST: Sometimes it just makes it easier to talk.

ANITA: (*voice dropping slightly*) I don't mean to be facetious. Don't get me wrong. I just really, I just really didn't want to have to go through it.

THERAPIST: (*pausing, and then softly*) It sounds like you've *really* been through the mill with everything so far. Is that right?

ANITA: Yes.

THERAPIST: Well, maybe we'll scrap getting to know each other. Maybe you can tell me where you would like to start.

ANITA: I really can't say. I'm sorry. As much as I've already said that I don't really want to go through the whole family history again, I honestly couldn't say where I would want to start. I am not the psychologist, so I don't really know what is actually relevant. So probably I was speaking out of place. But I really wanted you to know my feelings.

THERAPIST: It sounds like you have been through this many times. How many times have you been through it?

ANITA: I've lost count, (*pause*) but it's been all Sarah's life. The whole 13 years. I think the problems have varied, but they have been basically the same.

THERAPIST: What I would like to try and understand is why the help that has been offered you hasn't helped you so far. What has your experience been in trying to get help?

---

[2]The notation "==" within the transcript indicates interruption or talking over.

ANITA: Because we've been to so many different people who have told us so many conflicting things. I *am* going to have to go through it, I know. . . . You ask me why it hasn't helped. And I don't know. All I know is that I just feel like I've been alone. I haven't had a supportive family to start off with. Quite apart from that, I've just been totally confused by so many so-called professionals giving us their opinions, everything from food allergy to dyslexia.

THERAPIST: Of the people you have seen, have they been primarily supportive or unsupportive?

ANITA: (*pausing*) That's a difficult one to answer. I think that my opinion would be that they were doing a job.

THERAPIST: Did any of them seem to care about you as a person?

One doctor, said Anita, who had diagnosed her daughter as having food allergies, had displayed some concern. Of the number of therapists they had seen over the years, however, she believed that most were "reading from the textbook," and that her daughter was "just another kid among others." In her school, she was "just another number."

THERAPIST: Sarah, who do you think out of everybody that your family has seen, who do you think has been most supportive? Do you know what I mean by *supportive?*

DAUGHTER: Dr. M., I think. But he's hard to work out. He doesn't show what he's thinking.

THERAPIST: What do you think, Anita? Who in the rest of the world would be most supportive of you?

ANITA: Me.

THERAPIST: (*softly*) Is that right?

ANITA: Yes, I always have done (*voice dropping and eyes tearing*).

THERAPIST: When you say it always has been, does that mean just since you had Sarah, or that in terms of your whole life?

ANITA: Do I have to answer that?

THERAPIST: No.

DAUGHTER: At least make an attempt. I have to.

ANITA: OK. My whole life. But there's a lot Sarah doesn't know.

By this stage, the mother's initial negativity had lessened. For the duration of the interview, she spoke openly about her difficulties in her relationship with her ex-husband and her concerns about Sarah. The empathic exploration of her perception of mistreatment in the hands of professionals shifted her from her "resistant" stance.

On the one hand, the process of connecting with family members is simple and straightforward—talk to each person, appear warm and respectful, do not leave them waiting, avoid negative escalations. In practice, however, these small steps are often overlooked by therapists, and these parents are not forgiving. Having already had multiple negative interactions with professionals, they easily discount therapists as simply more of the same. What is novel and interesting to these parents is to discover a professional who genuinely seems interested in and respectful of them, and who even appears to like them.

Addressing Cultural, Racial, and Gender Differences

Therapists as professionals are, from the start, socially positioned differently from their working-class clients. The complexity of these differences is magnified when the clients are also of a less-dominant cultural extraction, racial origin, or sexual orientation than are their therapists. In these cases, it is important that the potential difficulties of the situation as experienced by the clients are anticipated by the therapist and brought into the conversation at an early stage. Although therapists of the dominant race/ethnicity may feel that working with a family different from them in race or ethnicity is not an issue for them, it may well be for family members, who experience the therapist as operating from stereotyped assumptions about them (Hall & Greene, 1994). By raising the issue early on, the therapist gives permission for these issues to be voiced and discussed and, in the process, becomes a person more worthy of the family members' trust. In doing so, the therapist must be prepared to hear and listen through the anger that may be just underneath the surface (Boyd-Franklin, 1989).

It is useful for white therapists to address the difference directly by asking family members how they feel about working with someone who is white. For example, African American clients are often sensitive to the "vibes" they sense as to whether they are being treated respectfully (Boyd-Franklin, 1989), and to microaggressions that is, the subtle way in which people of color are exploited, downgraded, or put down (Pinderhughes, 1990). Until assured of being treated respectfully, these parents may remain suspicious and on guard. By being able to directly address the issue of race and color, therapists are in a better position of correctly identifying *when* race is central to the presenting problem (Hardy & Laszloffy, 1994; Dyche & Zayas, 1995; Falicov, 1995).

Even in those situations in which the therapist is of the same subordinate group, it may be important for the therapist to ask family members how they feel about working with them, because the class difference between therapist and client may remain an issue. For example, a male African American therapist may be perceived as less streetwise and less masculine than his male clients, while the African American female therapist may be seen by her female clients as a (more successful) competitor and as seductive when she attempts to join with male clients.

In attempting to join with families of a minority culture, the therapist must be flexible in responding to the differences in expectations that different groups have of therapists. Treatment effectiveness with low-income African American clients appears to be clearly related to the ability of the practitioner to take a nonhierarchical stance and to join with clients as a peer and collaborator (Pinderhughes, 1990).

On the other hand, a more formal and authoritative stance may be taken when joining with Southeast Asian families, who expect the therapist to be an authority who interacts with them in a polite and formal manner (Lee, 1990). In such situations, the therapist is advised to use last names, correctly pronounced, and to respect traditional age–sex hierarchies. Different again are refugee families, separated from their family and culture, who may enter therapy with a yearning to connect with a therapist and the hope that the therapist will show genuine care and empathy. A therapist who exhibits warmth and concern is more able to win their trust (Lee, 1990).

Whenever a cultural or racial difference exists between therapist and family, the therapist must be prepared to adopt a learner, nonexpert role in allowing clients to educate him or her about the realities of their lives and the meanings the attribute to aspects of their culture (Pinderhughes, 1990). Knowledge about other cultures is invaluable; nevertheless, it should not take the place of allowing the particular family to tell their own story.

In eliciting from clients a description of their lives, therapists may often be presented with basic, material concerns over food, money, housing, and safety. When parents present one of these issues as a major concern, therapists may be able to engage families by helping them with some of these survival issues, and in doing so both increase their trustworthiness and create a more solid foundation for change in family relationships (Boyd-Franklin, 1989).

ESTABLISHING AND DEFINING CONFIDENTIALITY

Parents referred from the Department may fear speaking openly, concerned that information will pass from the therapist to the Department.

The issue of confidentiality is complex. On the one hand, we must be perceived as trustworthy in order to work effectively with the parents. On the other, at some stage, we may become alarmed about the safety of a child, our files could be subpoenaed to Court, or we might find agency policy determining our actions.

Some therapists attempt to resolve this dilemma by adopting a collegial approach with CP Workers and the Department. They remain totally open in giving information to other professionals and aligning themselves with the Department. In doing so, they reinforce the family members' perceptions that they are agents of the Department. Still other therapists adopt an adversarial role by aligning with the family, ensuring absolute confidentiality and ultimately conflicting with the Department. The way out of these difficulties is to have clearly defined criteria for what information will be shared with the Department and how it will be shared. It is generally important that the Department be aware of changes in the status of the case that will affect the likelihood of the child being at increased risk. On the other hand, parents need to experience therapy as a context in which they can reveal the most vulnerable aspects of themselves. In Table 6.1 we specify the information that is necessary to share with the Department. In Table 6.2 we outline the information that is generally unnecessary and unhelpful to share with the Department, unless this information has been discussed with the family, the parents have given consent for specific disclosures, and the particular purpose of the disclosure is clear.

It is imperative that the issue of when, how, and what information is shared between professionals be addressed during the initial meeting with the parents. While framing therapy as confidential, therapists need to present their criteria for having contact with the Department, explaining what type of information is or is not shared, and assuring parents that no contact with the Department will be made without their knowledge.

When it does appear necessary now or at some future date to share information with the Department, the reasons for doing so can be discussed with the parents, clearly explaining what is to be said. If the CP Worker telephones the therapist, it is important that, whenever possible, the parents are informed of the telephone call before the call to the CP Worker is returned.

TABLE 6.1. Information to Share with the Department

- Whether the family is proceeding with therapy or has dropped out.
- Whether the family is progressing or not in achieving the goals that the therapist and the Department have agreed upon.
- Whether the child is or is not currently at risk.
- Any new instances in which the child has been abused or neglected.

TABLE 6.2. Information the Therapist Is Not Obliged to Share with the Department

- Details of what is discussed in therapy.
- Personal information concerning the parents' past or marital concerns.
- Disclosures concerning abuse that occurred prior to the referral to therapy, assuming that, first, the child is currently safe and the Department has already investigated and intervened, and, second, that these disclosures do not seriously alter the ultimate goal or plan of therapy.[a]

[a]An instance where the goal of therapy might change, for example, is if sexual abuse is disclosed but only physical abuse had been suspected. In this situation, the Department would have to be informed.

The reason for upholding this principle is that it creates opportunities to earn the parents' trust. As described by one young mother, Lisa, trust develops gradually through a series of situations in which the therapist responds openly and consistently concerning every interaction with the Department.

THERAPIST: What has it been like for you to come here?

LISA: I've really enjoyed it, actually. At first I thought, "Oh, no, here we go again!" because we didn't really trust anyone, after what we have gone through. They go behind your back and write things down.

THERAPIST: What do you think made the difference in terms of you deciding you could trust me, after all that you've gone through?

LISA: Maybe because you wouldn't have anything to do with the Department unless you spoke to us first. We kind of felt like we could believe what you said. Like if they rung up, you'd always tell us and say to us, "Can I talk to them about this or about that?" Like you didn't ring them up and say to them, "Oh, guess what I know?" And you said you were working with us, not them. I think you can more or less tell when you can trust somebody. I guess it's just human nature, and I felt that; both of us did.

Without the parents' trust, therapy will be difficult if not impossible. Nevertheless, when there is a clear and immediate danger to a child, the therapist may be compelled to contact the Department first and inform the parents later. Although in many situations the therapist is better off enabling the parents to report the situation to the Department themselves (see Chapter 7), when this is not possible, the therapist's concern about the child's welfare must take precedence.

It is not in the parents' interests for their therapist to avoid contact with the Department. Worried CP Workers undermine therapy or break their agreements with parents when they are insufficiently reassured about the child's safety. Contact with the Department is necessary to describe to the CP Worker in detail any positive changes that have occurred in the relationship between the parent and child. Such details, however, should only be discussed with the Department after explaining the necessity of doing so with the parents and receiving their consent. In talking with any third person, such as a CP Worker, opinions should not be conveyed that are contrary to the opinions given to the parents. Consequently, in situations where there are concerns about the welfare of a child, it is wise for the therapist to be direct and honest with the parents about those concerns.

In the following brief example, we explain the nature of confidentiality and our relationship to the Department. Confidentiality was an issue for Julie, who said that she felt betrayed when her previous therapist had reported back to the Department concerning the content of the therapy sessions:

THERAPIST: Before you tell us your story about what happened to you, I think we should clarify for you how we work in relation to the Department.[3] As I said before, we are not part of the Department. When families come to see us because they have had difficulties with the Department or because they are worried about their child being hurt, it is often important for us to speak to the worker in the Department with whom they've had contact. Before we speak with anyone, however, we always tell parents that we going to do so, and we get the parents' consent for doing so. We tell the parents what we are going to discuss with the CP Worker, and we report back to the parents on the telephone call. We do not routinely report to the CP Worker, and we don't tell them all the details about the therapy. We think that it is important that you feel that you can talk openly with us. Do you have any questions about that?

JULIE: No, you've clarified things pretty well and clarified things with the Department. That was one of my main concerns, having gone through the other therapist. I found out that when you told him things, he relayed them back to the Department, and so I felt I couldn't really talk.

THERAPIST: Yeah. In our situation, if something came up that we were

---

[3]In many of the case examples that follow "we" refers to the therapy team. One of the therapists conducted the interview in the room, while the others observed behind a one-way screen. The person in the room who talks to the family is referred to as "the therapist."

concerned about with your kids, then we would talk to you about our concerns, and we would decide together what to do. Because we would expect that you would be concerned, too.

JULIE: Yeah. That suits me fine. The other therapist should have discussed it with me and listened to what I felt at the time. I felt that his reaction was wrong because he wasn't listening to what I was saying. I felt that he was judge and jury. And I didn't think that was his role. I thought his role was to talk to us and help us sort things out. Not to be judge and jury.

THERAPIST: How do you feel about proceeding then? Do you feel you would like to talk with us today?

JULIE: Yes, I feel like I want to go ahead.

THERAPIST: OK, maybe we should start. But if ever at any point you feel uncertain or worried about something you've said, you should feel free to say so to me. If anything should ever come up in the course of our conversation—or if you feel like we misunderstand. All right? So that we realize our errors.

JULIE: All right (*nodding her head*).

THERAPIST: What we would like to do today is that Kerrie will go behind the screen and I will stay here to talk with you, as I explained before. Is that all right with you if we do that now?

JULIE: Sure, of course.

Like Julie, Kurt and Sue, a young couple whose story is discussed in greater detail in the following pages, were also concerned about the issue of confidentiality in therapy because the previous therapist had reported back to the Department. According to Kurt, when he had admitted that one of the injuries to his infant may not have been completely accidental but was caused instead by his rough handling of her as he was dressing her, the previous therapist had passed this information on to the CP Worker. The Department was already aware of the other injuries to the child, and Kurt had admitted to causing them. Kurt believed, however, that the Department and the police now assumed that he had intended to hurt the child by twisting her arm. In the following example, we clarified that our contact with the Department would not be concerning any admissions of responsibility for previous situations, but rather would be confined to current concerns about the child.

THERAPIST: From our point of view, we would not feel any necessity to tell the Department about things you've done in the past. If you came in 2 weeks from now and you said, "I'm really stressed, I'm off my brain, I'm hitting my child," or "I'm afraid I'll hit my child," and "I can't control it," I'd say, "Kurt, we've got to do something about this." Because you both would be scared that you were going to kill her.

SUE: Oh, no, I wouldn't ever let that happen. I wouldn't let it go that far.

KURT: I would never let it go that far again. I would leave first.

THERAPIST: Of course, you wouldn't. We would all have to do something about it. That kind of thing does sometimes happen, and when it does, I talk to the parents about it. I don't do anything behind their backs. I would be open with you about anything that I was doing to protect you from hurting your child. But if you tell me something that happened before, and is not happening now, that's different.

KURT: They wanted the other therapist to find out what happened before.

Because the possibility always exists that files can be subpoenaed to Court, where parents may feel betrayed when the files' contents are revealed, notes written about the session have to remain consistent with the frame established with the family and not contain the therapist's transient frustrations and prejudices. It is also necessary to foreshadow the possibility that the Department will request a report for the Court at the conclusion of therapy. Instead of writing reports to the Department or to the Court, in many cases reports may be handled by writing the report in the form of a letter to the family which the parents can give to their solicitor and to the CP Worker. Letters will be explored in more detail in the following chapter.

GETTING THE STORY

The next item on the agenda for the initial meeting is to obtain the parents' account of how the family became involved with the Department and other professionals. There is another account that must eventually be elicited from family members that concerns the family's situation that led to the alleged abuse. In practice, these two accounts are often intertwined, and a focus on obtaining the first account inevitably reveals aspects of the second. We use the word "account" rather than the word "history," because we view information concerning the past as constructed in the present and influenced by the person's present interests and understood through the discourses in which the person operates. This is true of all information, whether it is received from the family, the CP Worker, or from other professionals. In this sense, the parents' account is no more or less credible than that of the CP Worker.

Obtaining the first account begins with the therapist asking the parents how they became involved with the Department and other professionals. The family's account of their involvement with professionals is explored for two reasons. First, it provides information about how the parents may respond to the therapist and, second, it demonstrates as great an interest in family members' definition of the situation as in the allegations of the referral source. Parents usually describe a sequence of events leading up to the allegations and subsequent interaction with the Department, the legal system, and other therapists. During this process, parents either acknowledge or deny the abuse. At this stage, the therapist does not focus on the abuse or the truth of the allegations but remains interested in the parents' relationship with the Department and other professionals.

Questions are addressed to all family members. Family members should experience the therapist as attentive, curious, interested, and empathetic to their distress and difficulties. Questions that appear to align the therapist with or against the Department are thus avoided. While actively soliciting interactional information in their construction of the problem, the therapist avoids siding with any one person or agency, or with any solution of the problem or description of events or individuals. It is important that the Department's opinion concerning the problem, or the way the Department defines the problem, not be accepted or represented by the therapist as "the truth." Where there seem to be differences in perceptions of the problem, events, or solutions within the family, questions are asked to elicit these differences. Questions concern the parents' and other family members' perceptions of (1) their initial contact with the Department and the evolution of their relationship with the CP Workers, (2) the Department's construction of the problem, and (3) the sequence of events leading to their arrival on the therapist's doorstep.

Eliciting such perceptions guides parents and encourages them to tell their account of what happened. The assumption that the therapist is an extension of the Department is also subtly challenged. By maintaining a focus on the relationship between the family and the Department, a space is created for the parents to begin to reveal aspects of their account of the abuse. When the parents are confused as to the Department's responsibilities (as is often the case with migrants and non-English-speaking parents), the therapist can also explain and clarify the Department's role and differentiate the Department's role from that of the therapist.

Toward the end of this section of the interview, the therapist offers to telephone the CP Worker to help clarify what the parents must do to reach their stated goal (e.g., return of a child). This discussion is outlined in more detail in the following chapter.

The following transcript is of Kurt and Sue revealing their involvement with the Department, the police, and their previous therapists. The interview creates space for the clients' discourse and demonstrates how an exploration of the first account (involvement with professionals and the Department) may lead the family to expose much of the second account (the situation concerning the alleged abuse), without the therapist risking engagement by questioning prematurely about the abuse.

CASE EXAMPLE: KURT AND SUE

Prior to the initial meeting, we received only brief information from the CP Department, the referring agency. Referral information included the names and ages of family members and the presenting problem, which was that Kurt had physically abused his 2-year-old stepson and his infant daughter, resulting in bruising and a fracture.

The family consisted of Kurt, 23; his partner, Sue, 22; their infant daughter, Jessica; and Sue's son from her previous relationship, Andy, now 3. The couple had been in a relationship for 2 years. During the first year, Sue had lived with Andy at her parents' home. The couple began living together a year later, prior to the birth of Jessica. Following the investigation by the Department, Sue had returned to live with her parents and younger brother. Sue's father was an executive for a large company, and their family home was located in a middle-class suburb. Kurt, on the other hand, was the youngest in a large working-class family. His parents were blue-collar laborers, and he had had only sporadic contact with them since he left home at 18.

When asked for their story about how they became involved with the Department. Kurt began the story by talking about how he received a call from his solicitor, who said, "The police want to charge you."

KURT: I said to him, "Do you know why I've got to go and see him?" And he said, "They want to charge you." I said, "Why? What's made them change their minds now? We've gone through everything with the Department because we want to get back together. We know we're all right, and all we need is to be left alone and given a fair go."

SUE: It's really hard with the Department, because everything goes in one ear and out the other. We've had three different CP Workers. I think I get really stroppy [irritable, hard to get along with] with them. And then we got Betty, and Betty's telling me that they could take my kids away from me and put them in a foster home. And I haven't even done anything to them, but they say they can't trust me about not going back to Kurt. Just because I'm trying to help him, they seem to think that that's all wrong.

KURT: Like the reason that we're not married is because when we met we were really in love and everything like that. But my brother and Sue's father had worked for the same company.

Kurt and Sue then told their story of how they met through Kurt's brother, Jim, who had worked as a foreman for Sue's father's company. Sue had been living at home with her parents at the time, and her mother was very involved in caring for Sue's son, Andy. A few months after Sue and Kurt became involved, Jim was fired from the company, a decision that he heatedly contested. Sue's father subsequently became aware that Sue was involved with Kurt and that Jim and Kurt were brothers. He pressured Sue to break up with Kurt. Sue and Kurt resisted breaking up and became secretive with their affair. Within a few months, however, Sue discovered she was pregnant, her parents again became aware of the relationship, and the couple became more determined to stay together. Against Sue's parents' wishes, they moved in together a few months before the baby was due.

As a semiskilled laborer, Kurt's work was often inconsistent, making his financial position precarious. To tide them over when Kurt was laid off, they borrowed money from Sue's parents. Kurt said he was upset, however, that her family seemed to think he was not good enough for Sue and encouraged her to separate from him.

KURT: I wanted her family to accept me, so I felt wanted. So we could get on as reasonable as possible without being childish about everything. Of course, things got worse since the first incident with Andy. Because there have been two incidents, the first time I did abuse Andy.

SUE: I wasn't there at the time. I asked Kurt to just mind Andy and Jessica while I went to my parents' house to get something. They were both asleep at the time.

KURT: I was tired, plus we'd had an argument earlier on that day. Well, she left me with the kids, and Jessica woke up screaming the minute she walked out, and she was just screaming and screaming, and there was nothing I could give her. And I tried to hold her and help her. Then, Andy woke up screaming. But he wouldn't let me pick him up. He just kicked and screamed, and then I started thinking, this is crazy, I shouldn't be thinking this way, and I jumped up and I slapped him. And as soon as I did I said to myself, "What are you doing?" and I tried to pick him up again and he just screamed. And I just thought, "God! look what's happening because of all this stupid stuff going on behind the scene."

Kurt then described how, when he realized how hard he had slapped Andy, he felt scared and shaken. He left the apartment and went out walking to "cool down." Sue was shocked and angry when she returned to find the two children alone and to see a hand mark across the toddler's cheek. She took Andy along with Jessica to the hospital. Meanwhile, Kurt had returned home to find Sue and the children gone. Within the next 48 hours, he was interviewed by both the Department and the police.

KURT: I just thought, this is incredible, this is such a nightmare!

THERAPIST: You must have been pretty scared by that time.

KURT: Well, the CP Workers started questioning us, and they just went over and over it. They kept Andy in the hospital. The next day, the police came and they came and charged me. I had to stay out of the place. Sue stayed home and I had to stay out.

SUE: I was really furious with Kurt after what happened. But then, after I talked to him, he was crying and everything, and when I was talking to him I realized we should have been communicating more and getting along better at that time, and that's more or less why I didn't leave him.

THERAPIST: What sense did you make of it, once you'd talked to Kurt. How did you understand it?

SUE: I was still really angry. I thought it was outrageous. I just said to him, "Why didn't you just leave the baby in one room and go out and shut the door?" That's what I would have done. The baby would have stopped screaming. Thinking back to it now, though, at that stage, Kurt was really, really stressed. He just had so much tension in his head, as if he could explode.

KURT: I just felt like we had to get away from everybody so that we could work out our own lives.

That day had been particularly tense, reported Sue, in that they had argued over extra work Kurt had turned down. Sue said she was worried about their income, which was totally dependent on Kurt's inconsistent work.

SUE: We didn't have much money then, and we were pretty worried about it, because we wanted things for the baby, and baby things cost a lot of money.

KURT: Can I just interrupt there. That's your point of view. I don't live for materialistic things, I don't worry about money. It's good to have money, but you know, some people have arguments and arguments over money. Back then, Sue used to worry too much about money, and I used to tell her not to worry.

Sue described how she found it hard to go from her own job and income (and one might hypothesize the security of her parents' home) to sudden dependence on Kurt. She was good at saving money; he was not. When the telephone bill came in, they had no money to pay it:

THERAPIST: Let me just take you back to your story. What happened after the police charged you?

KURT: Later on, well, the court date was set and the Department told us what to do.

SUE: We were meant to go to marriage counseling. Kurt was supposed to go on a stress management course and see a probation officer, and "the mother wasn't allowed to let the father see the children unsupervised." But they never did any of it, and then they turn around and tell us==

KURT: ==The court said that the Department was supposed to arrange all those things, but they never followed up on any of it.

SUE: They never got back to us. They just dropped the whole thing. The only thing they did follow up on was finding Kurt a stress management course.

KURT: And it was absolutely hopeless. It was no help at all. Just a room full of people supposed to be relaxing.

THERAPIST: So then what happened after that?

SUE: Well, when we went to court, the court said the children could stay with me, but only if I stayed with my parents, and Kurt could only have visits. This is just part of the whole deal.

KURT: I could only see Jessica and Andy once a week and only when the visit was supervised at Sue's place with her parents. Her family was really hard on me after doing it to Andy. They just couldn't accept me coming to their place. Jessica and Sue were living there, and it started to work up a grudge in me. I thought, "My daughter's over there, and they don't even want me in the place." I kept telling Sue, "I'm not very happy about this. It's really getting me down."

SUE: My Mom used to say, "You were living with a criminal. . . . Kurt is not Andy's father—he's a no-hoper." It just went on and on and got worse and worse.

KURT: Well, my grudge kept building up and I tried to talk to them once, but they sort of wouldn't talk, but it just kept getting worse and worse, and they kept talking behind my back, and that's when it starting getting between Sue and me. . . . A few weeks later, I was visiting for the afternoon and the baby had to be changed. I thought I could do it. I wanted to do it. But I was rough changing her clothes. I was having trouble. I said, "God damn jumpsuit," and I twisted her arm to get it through, and that's where I think it happened. I didn't even know, 'cause she was crying anyway because she wanted her bottle.

That night, Kurt asked Sue if there was anything wrong with Jessica's arm, believing that he might have dislocated the baby's shoulder. Sue had said, "Why would there be anything wrong with her arm?" Kurt did not say. She noticed when she changed Jessica that night that she had a "click" in her arm. Sue took the baby to a clinic, where the baby was diagnosed as having a broken arm, and the arm was set in plaster. The clinic phoned the Department, who contacted the police. When he was interviewed, however, Kurt maintained that it had been an accident:

KURT: So then the police came back into it. It all happened all over again, and they were saying, "Why hadn't you taken her to the hospital?" Instead of the baby clinic. And they were making up all sorts of things about it, saying that we had done everything all wrong.

SUE: We hadn't even heard of those kind of people who beat their kids. . . . All the things that happened from it. Kurt got a criminal record from it, and even having to go to all the courts.

THERAPIST: And what happened with the charge?

KURT: I got a 3-year bond for the first incident with Andy, and I have to see a probation officer once a month. At first, nothing happened about the baby's arm. It was only after we saw Marsha.

THERAPIST: Let me find out how you got to Marsha.

SUE: We were supposed to go to marriage counseling, and Kurt had to go to psychotherapy, and we had to see this counselor Marsha, and I guess in Marsha's report, which we haven't seen yet, she says that we still need a lot more counseling to work all these problems out.

KURT: So it's really the Department who was giving the judge ideas on how to make his decision. And the girl who's doing it from the Department doesn't like us, I'm sure. She just does not like us for some reason.

SUE: She used to say some terrible things to me on the phone==

KURT: ==And I used to get on the phone and have a go at her, and say "You're not allowed to talk to Sue like that."

SUE: She would just say, "You two will never be back together." And I used to say to her, "How do you expect to help us as a family if you're not interested in me or Kurt and you're only interested in Jessica and Andy, and you don't care if we get back together," and I would say, "On what basis does Kurt get to see Jessica?," and she would say, "We don't care if he does get to see Jessica." . . . So we went to the court in April, and then they prolonged it again until July, and then in that time we saw Marsha, the last counselor.

THERAPIST: What was it like seeing Marsha?

KURT: Well, she acted like she actually understood everything that we'd been through. And she said, "Even the best of families and the people who were most in love wouldn't have lasted through what you've been through." She understood. And after a few weeks I said, "There is one thing that we haven't said yet," . . . and she said, "What's that?" And I said, "Well, I was probably rough putting Jessica's jumpsuit on." And I told her how it happened and that I probably did do the damage. And she went and told the Department. She told them before we went to see them.

SUE: But I knew she had, because I got two phone calls within 5 minutes. One from Marsha and one from Betty [the CP Worker] and she said to us, "Well, I hear that you've got something to tell me."

THERAPIST: So when Marsha did that, how did that affect your relationship with her?

SUE: Well, at first we didn't worry about it, because it took 3 weeks before the police came. They keep telling us that the Department has nothing to do with the detectives, but it has. Betty must be in pretty close contact with them.

KURT: Well, so now the Department has told the police, and the police think that we were covering the whole thing up to begin with, so they are charging me again, 'cause now they don't think that it was an accident. They are making it out like—with Jessica—that I just grabbed her arm and twisted it, to break her arm. That's how they're putting it.

THERAPIST: So you think they're really misconstruing your intentions?

KURT: Yeah, yeah. And there's nothing we can do about it. They're saying I intentionally did it, but I know that's not so, and I know that and Sue knows that, but they're not believing us.

SUE: I think it's the fact that there are the two incidents, too.

THERAPIST: Did you decide to stop seeing Marsha or. . . . How was it you were referred on?

SUE: I didn't want to see Marsha again, because she would probably have to stand up in court against Kurt. She was really good to us, as if she really cared. But then she was being pushed to tell them what happened. I mean if you told her anything==

KURT: ==All we need is to be left alone instead of being sent to all these different people.

By the conclusion of this initial meeting with Kurt and Sue, we could hypothesize the pattern of interaction that had evolved between the couple, the Department, and previous therapists. There was also enough information to begin to hypothesize about the relationship context and levels of unfairness and oppression in which the abuse of the children was embedded. The following is a brief summary of these ideas.

On the one hand, Kurt and Sue described feeling invaded and controlled by the actions of the Department. On the other, although the Department's interventions had been extensive, the CP Workers appeared not to have followed through with many of the solutions proposed by the Department and the courts. The solutions that were followed up were not seen by Kurt and Sue as addressing the problem as they defined it. The high turnover of CP Workers meant that Kurt and Sue had little opportunity to work through conflicts and develop a trusting relationship. They perceived their CP Worker as trying to separate them, like Sue's parents, and this set them against her. They joined together in rebelling against both Sue's parents and the Department. It is possible that their oppositional relationship with the Department made it difficult for any CP Worker either to assess them adequately or be of assistance to them.

Although Sue and Kurt liked and trusted the therapist, Marsha, their increasing openness resulted in Kurt taking more responsibility for having hurt Jessica. This, in turn, resulted in a reactivation of intervention from the Department and the police, culminating, from Kurt's perspective, in his further punishment. From their point of view, an invisible, denied, yet very real connection linked the Department, therapists, and the police. It was important for us, as their new therapists, to take particular care in dealing with issues of confidentiality.

We suspected that any attempts by us to focus on problems in their relationship early in therapy would unite them against us, conveying to them that we might also be trying to split them up. Their recent crisis had, in any case, bonded them more closely, consequently minimizing the issues between them. The couple felt trapped and oppressed, and had no clear idea of what they needed to do to get the Department out of their lives. They knew neither how to resolve the problems that led to the abuse, nor how to reassure the Department that they had done so.

In describing their involvement with the Department, Kurt and Sue spontaneously provided some information concerning their account of the abuse. In particular, their account revealed aspects of how the abuse was connected to the gendered relations and material conditions of their lives. Kurt's and Sue's families stood in sharp contrast. Kurt was a blue-collar worker, as were his parents, whereas Sue's father's managerial position connoted greater income and status. This difference in status appeared to be at the basis of Sue's parents' initial rejection of Kurt. Kurt felt himself to be unfairly judged, and it was in this context that the couple's relationship began. The birth of the baby increased these tensions. The discourse of masculinity holds that Kurt's worthiness as a male is determined by his ability to earn and provide for his dependents. It was over his apparent failure in this area that he and Sue fought just prior to his striking his stepson.

On the one hand, the birth of Jessica solidified the bond between Kurt and Sue. On the other hand, it drew a wedge between them by casting them into traditional male and female roles. Having relinquished her own source of income, Sue was now dependent on Kurt's income and status. Exhausted and overwhelmed with an unequal share of domestic labor and with Kurt not living up to what she expected was his end of the bargain, Sue considered the situation unfair. Similarly, Kurt felt the situation to be unfair. Feeling abandoned by Sue, who was now preoccupied with the labor involved with the home and young infant, he resented the expectation that he work at a job he did not enjoy, particularly when the returns from the relationship were rapidly diminishing. Despite the apparently united front of this young couple, there remained the possibility that Kurt may have also physically abused Sue.

Although the situation became intolerable for both of them, Kurt could not easily face emotional separation from Sue. Disconnected from his own family and emotionally isolated in a work world of men, he had entrusted what he experienced as his deeper self to Sue and could not let go of her easily, particularly while feeling disconfirmed. Nor could Sue easily abandon Kurt while perceiving his vulnerability and dependence on her, and while experiencing some responsibility for her parents' rejection of him. By striking his stepson, Kurt effectively created a situation in which he and Sue had to physically separate but, importantly, not on Sue's parents' terms.

These hypotheses concerning the "account of the abuse" would be explored in later sessions. During this initial meeting, the focus was on the problems as Kurt and Sue defined them. They appeared to experience little hope of regaining control of their lives and had little faith that another professional could be trusted. In concluding the initial interview, we had to provide them with a different perspective.

BEGINNING WITH A POSITIVE FRAME

The initial meeting is ended by commenting on the underlying bonds of love within the couple or family and by summarizing how therapy may assist parents with the problem as defined by them. One aspect of this, as will be elaborated in Chapter 7, is an offer by the therapist to find out what exactly the CP Worker is requiring of the parents. The interview is concluded by offering the parents a choice about whether to commence therapy with this therapist, suggesting that the parents take some time to consider "whether we are the right people for you." Another appointment time is offered, which the parents can cancel should they decide to do so. In our experience, given this choice, parents generally decide to continue in therapy.

Kurt and Sue had identified two problems: the lack of support from Sue's family and the "intervention with no end" from the Department. In concluding the initial meeting with Kurt and Sue, the therapist commented on the couple's commitment to each other and their difficulties both with Sue's parents and the Department.

THERAPIST: Your love and your relationship has been seriously challenged several times in the last 2 years, and against all odds you have maintained your care and commitment.

First of all, you were challenged by your parents, Sue, who tried to break the two of you up. At a time when most couples look to their families for support in beginning a new relationship and a new family, you had none.

You were then challenged by the Department, which seemed to have little concern about the two of you getting back together and made it very difficult for you to know what you should do in order to get back together. You have been charged by the police, and there is also the threat of Kurt going to jail. Many young men in this situation would not have stayed around and risked being charged. Men who were less committed and devoted to their partners would have ran way and left the situation, and yet you, Kurt, have stayed.

There are very few people supporting you, and the help you have been offered by the Department seems to have set you back rather than help you to overcome these difficulties. Despite making many efforts, after months, you feel no closer to getting back together and putting the Department behind you than you were in the beginning.

KURT: That's right.

THERAPIST: We are interested in helping you find a way out of this situation. We would be happy to work with you if you think that we are the right people for you. You may need some time, however, to think about *whether or not* we are the right people for you.

KURT: I think it's worth starting.

THERAPIST: How about if we make an appointment for next week and then, if you are sure we are the right people for you to work with, we will start then. If not, you can cancel the session.

KURT: OK. What time? We'll come.

In ending the initial meeting, only those issues as defined by the parents are addressed. With Kurt and Sue, for example, we did not explore or comment on any of our hypotheses concerning the "account of the abuse," the exploration of which was reserved for later sessions. The therapist's initial goal is to create a context in which the parents can begin to trust. This means moving slowly and working toward resolving one of their initial concerns in order to deepen their trust.

Having obtained the parents' account of the involvement of the Department and other professionals, the Department's "account of the family" is now required. The next step is to make contact with the CP Worker. This must be done in a manner that does not breach the parents' trust in the therapist and that brings some clarity as to what the parents must do to resolve their difficulties with the Department. This next step is what will be elaborated further in the next chapter, where we will examine more closely the tripartite relationship between therapist, family, and protective services, and how therapists can prevent problems, intervene in difficulties, and assist parents in working toward goals set by CP Workers.

Working with "the Welfare" in Child-at-Risk Cases

ONCE the parents have been engaged through an initial meeting, the therapist's next challenge is how to position him- or herself in relation to child protection authorities. Unlike many other referral sources, CP Workers frequently maintain an interest in the family long after making a referral to therapy, and they wield significant power in determining whether a child or parent remains with or is able to return to the family. Parents frequently perceive them as foe rather than friend. Complicated relationships may develop between therapists, who perceive the situation from the parents' viewpoint, and CP workers, who must ensure the safety of the child. In this chapter, we discuss how the therapist can be positioned as power broker when working at the interface of the interaction between the CP Worker, the parents, and the therapist.

The significance of the relationship between the therapist and CP Worker in determining the outcome of therapy was brought home dramatically to us early in the therapy project when working with Maria Reynolds, a single-parent mother of three children, and with her son, Christopher, 11. Maria had been on her own since leaving her last partner a few years before, after several years during which she and the children suffered from his violent outbursts.

Maria and her children were ordered by the Court to attend family therapy after the Department had placed Christopher in temporary foster care. In making the referral, the CP Worker explained that Christopher had run away from home after being beaten by his mother. When the Department had contacted his mother, Maria said she did not want Christopher at home because he was beating up his younger brother. When I asked the CP Worker what needed to happen for the Department to allow Christopher to return home, she replied that "Maria would have to want Christopher home, and Christopher would have to want to go home."

As I worked with this family over the next few weeks, it became apparent that Christopher, the eldest, was jealous of his younger brother's close relationship to their mother and angry with the middle brother's misbehavior, which the mother was unable to control. When put in charge of his brothers as his mother retreated into depressed withdrawal, he felt unable to manage and attempted to physically put his brothers in their place. As Maria better understood Christopher's behavior, she reached out to Christopher, they both cried, and the emotional wall between them came down. Christopher, his mother, and brothers all said they now wanted Christopher to return home. No longer perceiving Christopher to be at risk, I also wanted him home so that I could continue to work with them as a family. After this session, I made this suggestion to the CP Worker, who said she was skeptical that any change could take place so quickly and that Christopher could not return home immediately.

When Maria and her children, minus Christopher, showed up for their appointment 2 weeks later, Maria told me that in the intervening 2 weeks, the CP Worker had not allowed her to visit Christopher at the scheduled visitation time. When the CP Worker did not arrive with Christopher, I telephoned and she told me that she was arranging for the permanent placement of Christopher into foster care. When I objected, the CP Worker accused me of being only on the side of the mother. She maintained that Christopher was afraid to go home and that Maria needed at least 2 years of individual therapy before any changes could be expected.

Aware of the CP Worker's intentions only a few days before the Court date, I hastily presented the Reynolds family's case to a Legal Aid lawyer, who represented Maria at the Court a few days later. As a result, the Magistrate rejected the CP Worker's proposal and, instead, ordered that temporary care continue and that the family continue in family therapy. I was relieved until told by Maria a few days later that Christopher had been placed with a family in the extreme western suburbs, a journey for Maria of 4 hours round-trip by public transport. I also received a strange call from a family therapist in another agency, announcing that she was now the therapist for the Reynolds family's case. I arranged through the mother's lawyer to have responsibility for the therapy returned to me, but we could do nothing about the location of the placement.

What struck me most in this case was that there were several points at which Maria, the mother, could have objected to the Department's procedures but did not and, instead, adopted a passive and powerless position. Had I not advocated on Maria's behalf, she most certainly would have lost her son. I was also struck by the apparent disjunction between my image of the CP Worker—the single, childless professional—and this mother, Maria, who was older, a mother of three, a refugee from men's violence now living with her children in poverty.

The CP Worker had no interest or incentive to really understand Maria. Possibly, neither did Maria with regard to the CP Worker, but the CP Worker held the power to define the situation. Maria was the CP Worker's *other*. She was everything the CP Worker was not: working class, poor, uneducated, apparently callous with her children.

Why did Maria Reynolds so easily adopt a powerless position in the face of what I perceived to be injustice? Why, after working successfully in therapy with me, had Maria not even thought to inform me or seek my help when the CP Worker first refused to allow her to visit Christopher?

While I had for some time considered myself a feminist, Maria and women like her did not recognize themselves in me. I was privileged, a white, middle-class professional whose life at every turn held options and opportunities never afforded Maria. This was an uncomfortable position for me. Without my intention or control, my social position and my professional status cast Maria into the position of being my *other* (Mac-Kinnon, 1993). Despite her apparent trust of me during the therapy sessions, Maria could only expect that in the end, I would align against her, that despite our apparent difficulties, the CP Worker and I were part of the same professional discourse, a discourse that she did not understand or ever have much hope of negotiating successfully within.

Maria's story taught us that the relationship between parents and the CP Department cannot be left to chance or goodwill. Nor can we take for granted how we will be perceived by either of them. The relationship between the therapist and the CP Worker, and between the CP Worker and the parents, must be considered an intrinsic part of the therapy.

The approach described in this chapter was conceived with the following objectives in mind: First, we sought to negotiate workable presenting problems that would be acceptable to both CP Workers and parents and would eliminate no-win situations and never-ending intervention. Second, we aimed to decrease parents' perceptions of therapists as an extension of the Department and as taking the CP Workers' side against them, without minimizing the abuse or underestimating the risk to the child. This entailed finding alternatives to the ways therapists traditionally communicate with and report to child protection professionals and the Courts. Third, we aimed to address those situations in which we perceived CP Workers as acting inconsistently or unfairly and those in which conflictual relationships between CP Workers and parents locked parents into postures that confirmed the CP Workers' negative perceptions of them.

ESTABLISHING A WORKABLE RELATIONSHIP WITH CHILD PROTECTION PROFESSIONALS

Although it is essential to not appear to parents to be on the side of CP Workers, it is also necessary to engage and develop rapport with CP Workers, understand their construction of the problem and expectations of therapy, and liaise between the family and CP Worker in order to establish workable objectives for therapy.

Recall that when a family was referred from the Department, only minimal information was obtained from the CP Worker making the referral, and an arrangement was made to call back after the meeting with the family. During the first interview, the therapist then discusses with the parents the possibility of contacting the Department to find out what changes would enable the CP Worker to consent to the parents' stated goal (e.g., return of the child or return of the parent to the family). A section of an interview with Kurt and Sue, whose story was described in greater detail in the previous chapter, illustrates how this was done.

Kurt and Sue had been living apart for several months, since Kurt had been charged with assault of his stepson Andy. Kurt and Sue had repeatedly said throughout their "initial meeting" that (1) they wanted to get back together, and (2) they wanted the Department to leave them alone. In seeking permission to speak with the CP Worker, the therapist referred to these goals.

THERAPIST: One of the worst things right now is that you don't really know how to get out of the situation you're caught in. You keep going around and around, without any direction or any idea of how to make this situation end.

KURT: No, we can't make any plans now. It's just all up in the air.

THERAPIST: What I sometimes find helpful with this sort of thing is for me to speak with your CP Worker to see if I can get a list of things that *she thinks* that you have to do in order for the Department to leave you alone to live your life.

SUE: Well, whenever we tell her anything she just says, "Yeah, yeah, well lots of people go through those kinds of problems."

THERAPIST: Well, what I could do is to say to her, "OK, well, we need to have some goals," and to get her to be specific with me about the kinds of things you need to do in order to reassure her that you can be left alone.

SUE: What kinds of things do *you* think that we need to do to reassure her?

THERAPIST: We need to find out what *she's* thinking, so that we have something concrete to work toward. And that will give us some sort of direction, some sort of goal that we know we can achieve. So that she's going to be more assured that things are OK. Because as it is, if it's just sort of "go to counseling," you could be caught in a never-ending circle. (*Sue and Kurt nod.*)

SUE: That's how we feel.

THERAPIST: I don't know what she'll say, but sometimes when I talk to CP Workers I can get them to be more specific, so we actually have something concrete that you know that you can do.

KURT: Yeah, well we've been apart for 8 months now and there's nothing to look forward to, because I don't know what's happening. I think that the only way to help us is for us to get back together, and then when we come up against these problems is for us to talk to you.

THERAPIST: Well, I agree with that, so I guess what we have to do is work on enough things here that we can reassure Betty that you can get back together. Then we can actually deal with some of those problems as they arise. (*Kurt nods.*) (*pause*) How would that be, then, if I telephoned Betty to see if I could get her to be more specific about what you have to do?

SUE: Sure. But let me tell you, she's a strange person.

After obtaining the parents' consent in this way, the CP Worker is recontacted and engaged in a longer discussion that has four specific purposes. The first aim is to uncover CP Workers' construction of the problem and their attempts to intervene thus far. This includes exploring their perception of their relationship with family members, including their view of each parent's response to intervention. The second aim is to uncover CP Workers' implicit and explicit expectations of the therapist. For example, CP Workers frequently hope that therapists will confirm that the parents are abusive, change the problem quickly or change particular family members, obtain evidence that will enable them to decide the outcome of the case or to provide the court with information, or provide a particular type or style of therapy.

Once CP Workers' concerns and expectations are fully explored, the third aim is to have CP Workers experience the therapist as understanding their position and empathizing with their difficulties in managing the case. The fourth aim is to assist CP Workers in specifying changes in family members' behavior that would be evidence that the problem has changed and that the parents are ready for their stated goals (e.g., for the CP Worker to end her visits). Normally, CP Workers are able to provide answers to these questions only through careful questioning, and direction from the therapist and the therapist must allow the same time and attention to these discussions as are given to family interviews.

Rather than "collaborating" with CP Workers in the traditional sense, CP Workers' views are not privileged over those of the parents. Rather, CP Workers and the parents are viewed as operating within differing discourses. The perspective of the participants within these discourses has real effects in terms of how each person behaves and, thus, in terms of their effects on others.

Finally, it is explained to the CP Worker that the next step is to seek the parents' response to the proposed objectives. In doing this, the therapist conveys that he or she is negotiating on behalf of the CP Worker to obtain the parents' agreement to these objectives which, once accepted, become the goals of therapy. It is critical to the success of therapy that this conversation with the CP Worker is immediately followed up with a letter addressed to the CP Worker that summarizes the proposed objectives.

Creating Objectives

In the subsequent telephone call with Betty Smith, the CP Worker for Kurt and Sue, the therapist initially elicited Betty's story about the family and the abuse of their child.

Betty's "account" can be briefly summarized as follows: The assault of Andy, Kurt's stepson, followed by the injuries to the baby, left Betty extremely concerned about Kurt ever being left alone with a child. Kurt was "possessive and demanding of Sue's attention." He was jealous of Andy and had found it "difficult to cope" when the baby was born, a difficulty related to his "early relationship with his mother." Sue appeared to be rebelling against her parents. She did not seem to "take seriously" the injuries that Kurt had inflicted on the baby and appeared to be more interested in protecting him than the baby. Sue was "getting railroaded by Kurt" and "enjoyed taking Kurt's side in blaming others." Kurt handled the baby "too roughly" during his supervised access visits and seemed to have little sense of how to manage young children. Kurt had not acknowledged the seriousness of the injuries to Andy and Jessica, nor his "responsibility" for inflicting them. He seemed "magically to believe that he could simply decide not to do it again." Betty's attempts to convince him otherwise had proved fruitless. The relationship between the couple and the CP Worker had deteriorated to the point that Kurt and Sue had refused to speak with Betty.

Betty explained that the couple were to return to Court in 6 weeks' time, and, until then, Kurt was allowed access visits with Jessica while under the supervision of Sue's mother. Betty indicated that it was unlikely that the Court would change these conditions given the Department's ongoing concern about the safety of the child and the seriousness of the injuries.

In discussing with Betty her perceptions and concerns, we were able to elicit from her four behavioral objectives, which, if fulfilled, would enable Betty to take steps toward allowing the family to reunite. Following the telephone call, we sent the following letter to Betty, outlining the discussion and listing the four behavioral objectives:

Dear Ms. Smith,

This is to summarize our telephone contact on concerning Sue F. and Kurt T. You expressed your concerns about Andy and Jessica given the seriousness of Jessica's injuries. You want to ensure that before returning to both parents, the children will be safe. The objectives you propose for therapy (i.e., steps that Sue and Kurt can work toward as a way of achieving their goal of reuniting as a family) are as follows:

1. Kurt and Sue must acknowledge that the injuries to Andy and Jessica were serious. Therapy must explore the situation that led to these injuries.

2. Kurt must demonstrate that he is aware of how he injured Jessica, and that he has alternative means of coping with difficult feelings in a stressful situation.

3. Kurt must demonstrate that he can handle a young child gently and has empathy for the child's needs and feelings.

4. Sue must be prepared to protect the children from further injury, even if this means having to confront Kurt or separate Jessica from Kurt. Sue must demonstrate that her first concern and priority is the safety of the baby, and her second concern is maintaining the family unit.

I hope this accurately summarizes our conversation. If any of these details are incorrect, would you please call me so that we can change them. In the meantime, I will forward a copy of this letter to Sue and Kurt, and discuss with them these goals and ways they can begin to work toward achieving them.

Yours sincerely,

Laurie MacKinnon,
Family Therapist

Because Betty had perceived the couple very negatively, eliciting her concerns and transforming these into clear objectives was an extensive but straightforward process. There are situations in which CP Workers are less concerned than we expect they should be in the circumstances or in which we perceive their suggestions for objectives as too easily met. This would be the case, for example, in a situation of sexual abuse in which a CP Worker is unsure of what changes the parents could make, or is prepared to allow a father to return home before we believe it might be safe to do so. In such situations, the therapist can make suggestions throughout the discussion with the CP Worker, and the discussion culminates in objectives that might, in fact, more accurately reflect the therapist's notion of objectives, but which the therapist can attribute to the CP Worker.

Letters as "Contracts" and "Reports"

Letters form the backbone of our therapy in child-at-risk cases. Telephone discussions or meetings with CP Workers are immediately followed up with letters summarizing the therapist's understanding of the discussion. The high turnover rate in child protection work frequently means that the CP Worker who begins a case is not the one concluding it. By writing letters, therapists make productive use of a bureaucratic rule of the Department (i.e., all correspondence must be placed in the file). Consequently, letters are available to subsequent CP Workers, who are thus oriented to the direction of the case and are more likely to remain committed to the agreements previously made.

These letters also form the basis of subsequent "reports" concerning the changes occurring in the family over the course of therapy. "Reports" are written as letters addressed to the family and, referring back to the objectives, state, for example, that "the objectives for your therapy as outlined by the CP Worker were as follows: . . . We have perceived you working toward these objectives in the following ways: . . . ." This helps to ensure that the CP Worker adheres firmly to the decisions made with the therapist and lessens the likelihood of the CP Worker unilaterally changing direction without discussion with the therapist. Ultimately, letters are a contract between the parents and the CP Worker. They provide hope for the parent in that there is some way out of the current situation, and reassurance for the CP Worker in that changes are occurring to ensure the child's safety.

Last, such a "contract" for therapy means that the CP Worker, rather than the therapist, identifies the issues to be explored. The therapist can thus avoid two common pitfalls: either evading the very issues for which the family is referred in order to ensure that the parents continue in therapy, or, alternatively, confronting the parents and thus confirming the perception that the therapist was aligned with the CP Worker.

In returning to the situation of Kurt and Sue, during the second session, the therapist provided the parents with a copy of the letter to the CP Worker and read out the list of behavioral objectives.

SUE: So how is all that going to be done? Mainly through counseling, I guess, is it?

THERAPIST: Well, I think there are some that things we have to look at. For instance, even if we achieve these things, how will Betty know we have?

KURT: She's always said those things to us from the beginning. Just what you've read there. And we've said, "OK, Betty, but what do you want me to do? I'm doing everything I can."

THERAPIST: Well, I have a few ideas about how we can approach this, and you probably have some ideas, too. For instance, let's just take the easiest ones first.

The therapist read through each of the CP Worker's conditions and suggested how some of the objectives could be achieved through therapy.

THERAPIST: For instance, let's take number 3, that you must be able to *demonstrate* handling a young child. Well, you could bring Andy and Jessica to the session, and you could play with them and deal with them here. We could talk about different ways of managing children and the needs of young children. (*Kurt nods.*) I could talk to Betty about what we've done, and I could also write a letter saying how I've seen you interact with her.

SUE: Well, sometimes parents have differences of opinion. Like I might say it should be one way, Kurt might say it should be another, so we could talk about some of those different ways here.

The parents began to refer to some of their differences in terms of handling the children.

SUE: Even things like, if you put Kurt and me back together right now, and Kurt said anything to Andy to discipline him, Andy would just come running to me, because he doesn't spend much time with Kurt, and he doesn't know him very well. So things like that could cause problems, too.

The issues identified by the CP Worker and the subsequent behavioral conditions do not necessarily reflect the therapist's assessment of the situation. They simply provide a framework within which the parents can experience hope and perceive the therapist as acting as their advocate. Family members begin to address areas they might otherwise prefer not to, and therapists might begin to work on issues they judge to be relevant.

Although "contracts" between CP Workers and parents are a useful beginning in shifting an otherwise adversarial relationship, sometimes they are not sufficient to effect a change in the stereotypes each hold of the other, stereotypes that have been reinforced through multiple negative interactions. In order to enable CP Workers to perceive positive changes in parents who to them appear only hostile and "different," it may be necessary to intervene in the CP Worker–parent relationship.

INTERVENING IN THE CP WORKER–FAMILY RELATIONSHIP

Because the relationship between CP Worker and parents, whether positive or negative, inevitably affects the process and outcome of therapy, therapists require an interactional understanding of their relationship based on each person's perception of the interaction.

Returning to the situation of Kurt and Sue, for example, the early interviews with the couple and our discussions with the CP Worker were both filled with negative comments of the other, as is evidenced in the following excerpt:

KURT: I think Betty's younger than me, probably about 21 or 22. All she can seem to come up with after we talk to her, and after everything we do, is to say that "what happened with Andy and Jessica is a bad thing." And we know that, but what are we trying to do here? All she can say is "But, but, but," and I say, "Is it going to go on until we're 80," hearing "But, but, but"?

SUE: Once she got me so upset I screamed and swore at her.

KURT: Sue lost her temper at her.

SUE: And she just sat there like this (*crosses her arms and looks stern*), staring at me.

KURT: And then she used that as evidence in saying that Sue can't control herself. They drive you to that point. They drive you to the point where you could do anything!

The pattern of interaction between this couple and the CP Worker was an escalating conflict in which the CP Worker behaved in a controlling and critical manner and the parents, in turn, were defensive, angry, and rejecting. Once we understood their interaction, we had the choice of working through the parents to change the relationship or of holding a joint meeting.

Coaching the Parents

The essential factor in coaching parents to behave differently toward the CP Worker is providing the parents with an alternative understanding of the CP Worker's behavior. The therapist must be able to use culturally relevant explanations and metaphors in a language that the parents can understand. Having identified the pattern of interaction between Sue and Kurt and their CP Worker, Betty, we began to coach them to behave differently toward Betty in their next meeting. We created the frame that the parents were "caught in a catch-22" in which their actions confirmed to Betty that they were "child abusers" and thus elicited the very behavior they so disliked from Betty.

The creation of this frame began early in the interview by the therapist asking hypothetical questions in relation to the fourth objective (which was that Sue demonstrate that her first priority was the safety of the children). "What would happen," asked the therapist, "if despite all the years of therapy and help, Kurt was still intolerant of children and had a very short fuse, and therefore Andy and Jessica were still at risk with him?" Sue answered that she would leave Kurt to try to bring him to his senses. The therapist continued, "What if you found that Kurt would not get help or that help would not change him at all? What would you do then?" Sue answered that she would leave him and take the children with her. Kurt added that if he were in such a situation again, he would "leave for at least 3 months." Sue then described how she had told the previous CP Worker that if the situation deteriorated, she was prepared to leave Kurt and not allow Kurt to see Jessica. However, when Betty, the current CP Worker, had demanded that Sue repeat the statement, Sue argued with her, deciding that "I would never give Betty the pleasure of hearing it from me."

SUE: She wanted me there and then, on the spot, to tell her, and I'm kind of really stubborn. So I got really cranky with her.

THERAPIST: My hunch is that if Betty could actually hear you say it, it would make a big difference to her. Because her fear would be that if things got bad again, that you would let Kurt hurt Andy or Jessica.

SUE: But I wouldn't.

THERAPIST: I know you wouldn't. But I think she's afraid that you would always make excuses for Kurt and wouldn't actually leave him if the children were at risk again. In terms of what we can do to reassure Betty about number 4, it might be important at some point for you to talk to her. You might want to do that by yourself, or we might want to invite her to the session. . . .

Kurt was caught in the same symmetrical interaction with the CP Worker as Sue. Although he acknowledged to us his concern and responsibility for having injured the children, he refused to do so with the CP Worker. His refusal to do so made it even less likely that the CP Worker would be able to perceive any positive changes that resulted from therapy.

THERAPIST: Did you ever hear that phrase, "catch-22"?

KURT: Yeah.

THERAPIST: Well it came from a story about this guy who wanted to get out of the army, but the only way he could get out was to prove that he was crazy. But if he went crazy in the army, he was normal, because the army drove everybody crazy. So, in other words, there was no way out of it. (*Kurt and Sue both smile.*) And I think that's partly what's happened to you. You've got caught in a catch-22. The CP Worker basically says to you that you have to show that you're upset about what happened and that you acknowledge that you abused Jessica. But the trouble is that if you acknowledge that you abused your child, *you think* she is going to say, "Well, if you're a child abuser, then you shouldn't have your child back."

KURT: Well that's exactly what I think. If I say that, she's going to think that I'm still like that now.

THERAPIST: That's right, so you're caught in a catch-22.

KURT: Yeah.

THERAPIST: So when you try to say to her, "Look, everything's OK now, we can get back together now." Then she says, "Ah ha! He doesn't really acknowledge that he abused his child. Of course, child abusers never admit that they abused their child."

SUE: (*Laughs.*)

KURT: Yeah.

THERAPIST: So we have to figure out a way to demonstrate to her that you and your situation have changed. We have to figure out a way to get out of the catch-22, to show her that she no longer has to be worried about you. Because right now, when you try to reassure her that she does not have to be worried, it makes her more worried.

SUE: Uh huh.

KURT: Yeah, I know. That's how I see it, too. You feel like you're wasting time going and talking to her, because you feel like you don't get anywhere. There's nothing I can do. All I know is that when I'm with Andy and Jessica now, how I think and how I feel is completely different to how I felt back then.

THERAPIST: (*to Kurt*) I think that as long as she sees you as trying to hurry up the process, she's going to keep putting on the brakes, thinking that you're not taking it seriously.

KURT: Yeah.

THERAPIST: Well, I think there's something that you can do about that. I don't know if either of you could do it right now, because you've been pushed around a lot. The most important thing right now is that you not fight with Betty. (*pause*) When you read stuff in the newspaper about child abusers, what do you think they're like?

SUE: Rough.

KURT: You get a bad image of them.

THERAPIST: So what does the bad image look like?

KURT: A drug addict that doesn't love their children. Worries about themselves a lot. Drinking.

THERAPIST: How do you think a child abuser would react to a CP Worker?

KURT: Well, I think a lot of child abusers couldn't stand to be told how to treat their children, even though they couldn't handle them.

SUE: They wouldn't take anything from a CP Worker. I think they'd get all heated up about it.

THERAPIST: See, my theory is that a lot of CP Workers have that same view of child abusers. Now you two don't look to me like the kind of child abusers you were describing, but I bet you that when you get heated and stubborn, and get into fighting with the CP Worker, she thinks that you're acting like child abusers. Because she would think that child abusers are nasty, angry people who don't listen, and so on. (*Sue nods and laughs.*) Now I know if I was in your situation, I would feel just as angry as you, and I would have a hard time of it too. But I think the thing is, the more that you argue with her, the more she thinks, "Ah ha! They really *are* child abusers!"

KURT: Yeah (*smiles*).

SUE: Kurt's not as bad as me. It's me, really, who argues with her.

THERAPIST: So I think what we have to look at is how the two of you keep convincing her that you are child abusers. (*Sue nods and laughs.*) Because she doesn't know you very well and doesn't get a chance to get to know you well, all she sees is anger. She doesn't get to see you as people. . . . We have 4 weeks before you have to go back to the Children's Court. Even if we made a lot of changes over the next month, I doubt there is very much we could do to convince Betty in that time that you'd be ready to get back together.

KURT: No, she wouldn't think it was long enough.

THERAPIST: Which means that there's not much we can do about it before then. My hunch would be that the best way that we could convince her that you understand the seriousness of what has happened and that you have changed would be if the two of you were to go to Betty and say that as a result of coming here, you realize that there is a lot you want to work on, that you don't think you are ready to get back together in 4 weeks, and that you would like to have a couple of more months after the court date in order to come to counseling and to take a parenting course. And then ask her if she has a parenting course she would recommend. (*Both Sue and Kurt nod slowly.*) If they're not going to let you get back together in July, then I think that the best way is to beat them to the punch. Instead of waiting for them to tell you that you can't do it, you say, "We don't want to get back together yet, because we need more time in therapy." And they would say, "What! We've never heard this before! These people aren't acting like normal child abusers!" Then you start to get out of that image, and they can start to think of you as just two young people who've been under a lot of stress. They start to get a different picture of you, and that, I bet, would be a start to getting out of this catch-22. (*pause*) (*Both Sue and Kurt nod.*) Do you think you could do that?

KURT: Sure.

THERAPIST: I think we should realistically set our goals for you getting back together for something like 4 months. That gives us enough time to work through these points that Betty has made and find ways of reassuring her.

KURT: OK.

SUE: Sure.

In this situation, we coached Sue and Kurt to behave in a way that was different from the stereotyped expectations that the CP Worker had developed of them through their interaction with her. This allowed for the emergence of a different type of relationship between the CP Worker and the couple. During the fourth interview, the couple reported that they had met with Betty and told her that they needed more time in therapy. They had also asked her advice about parenting classes.

THERAPIST: What did you say to her exactly?

KURT: Well, she asked me, like about 2 minutes after we arrived, "How's everything going, like?" And I said, "Oh, good, no problem." The first therapy lesson was a bit of an experience, but after that, we settled down and relaxed and all that. And we think that after the court, we'd like to give it another 3 months or so and maybe take some parental classes and that. Just to make sure that we are ready.

THERAPIST: And what was her reaction?

KURT: She said, "Oh, yeah, that sounds good." Well, Sue had already told her about it, and she said, "Good for you. I'll try and get it organized." But she seemed a lot more pleasant (*glances at Sue, who nods*).

THERAPIST: And how did she seem to you when you told her?

SUE: Well, I first spoke to her on the telephone when I told her, and she seemed pretty happy.

KURT: She seemed to be more at ease toward us after I told her. I sort of had the feeling, you know, like how you were saying last week, that she had sort of thought that we were rushing it and not taking it seriously. And I think she has relaxed a lot more now.

THERAPIST: So it might have changed how she saw you a bit, instead of seeing you as child abusers.

KURT: Yeah, more as buddies.

SUE: Kurt was playing with Jessica and Andy, and I was talking to her the whole time during the visit.

KURT: I made a sort of joke afterwards and said to Sue, "Well, why don't you invite her around for lunch?"

THERAPIST: Boy, would that blow her mind! (*Kurt and Sue laugh.*)

SUE: Yeah, she was pretty all right yesterday.

The shift in the relationship between the parents and CP Worker was significant but tenuous. In order to highlight the importance of Kurt and Sue maintaining a positive relationship with the CP Worker, these relationship changes were explored in detail. Hypothetical questions were asked concerning the future of the relationship as a way of increasing the parents' awareness of their potential to contribute to the outcome of the interaction between themselves and the Department. By having the couple rate their relationship with the CP Worker on a 10-point scale, the therapist developed with them a shorthand method of referring to the quality of the interaction. This allowed the therapist in each subsequent session to inquire about their relationship with the CP Worker, comparing it again on the 10-point scale.

THERAPIST: If she was here, how do you think she would say she saw the two of you yesterday?

KURT: Probably a lot more as parents than as child abusers. More as a family. Before, I used to do something and I'd feel tense all over, and yesterday I felt all right==

THERAPIST: ==Well, let's say if we were to look at your relationship with Betty, say, before last week, if 10 was really positive and zero was really negative, where was it before last week?

KURT: Well, it changed. It went up and down. But probably between 3 and 4.

SUE: Well, if you took it back to the last court case, it would have been zero, because then everybody had a grudge against everybody, and she had a grudge against==

KURT: ==I had a grudge against her because she was interfering.

THERAPIST: So it's come up from zero to 3 to 4, and how would you say it is now compared to before?

KURT: I put it around, uh, 8.

THERAPIST: *Eight?* Really!

SUE: Well, you just need to know how they think!

KURT: Right. They can be nice to you, but they can be completely different.

Sue mentioned that the CP Worker had inquired about Sue moving from her parents' home to living on her own for a while with the children. She interpreted this as the CP Worker's increasing openness to the idea of Sue eventually moving back with Kurt.

THERAPIST: How do you think she's thinking differently about you, that she would ask you about that?

SUE: Well, she might trust us a lot more.

THERAPIST: In order to convince Betty that you're not child abusers, and that you're normal parents who love their children, where do you think you would need to maintain your relationship with her on that scale of 1 to 10?

KURT: Probably 8 or 9. Couldn't get much further.

SUE: Well, I'm sure that she was a lot more pleasant yesterday, because she even said to me, "Sue, if you want more visits down here for you and Kurt, I'll do them." So she must have been enjoying herself more than before.

THERAPIST: What do you think would need to happen to get your relationship to change from a 6 or an 8 to a 9?

KURT: It's hard to say. It might take time, like for us to attend the parenting classes.

SUE: Yeah, I think that she has to see that we're trying to do everything that we can.

KURT: Back then, 7 or 8 months ago, we were pretty harsh and we had, like, a sort of a wall between us. So now I think she is just waiting to see if anything like that comes up again.

THERAPIST: So it sounds like things are good now and it's more a matter of time, and if you can keep the relationship with her the way you have it now, that she will trust you more.

KURT: Yeah, like if we just said, "Forget it, we aren't going to therapy anymore," she would say, "Oh, well, back to zero."

THERAPIST: Do you think that she likes you more as people now?

KURT: Oh, yeah, I think so, yeah. Just the way she sort of says things like "Hello" and that.

SUE: She's more of a friend, that's what I said. (*laughs*) She didn't argue with me as much. We talked about things with Jessica and how I should look after her and stuff. And she told me that she thinks I've done a marvelous job with Andy, and she said that he was a credit to me, and like I had this problem with my mom telling me what Andy should eat, and Betty said, "Don't worry about what your mom says. You do what you think's right, and if she gives you any trouble, I'll talk to her."

THERAPIST: Backing you up.

SUE: Yeah.

THERAPIST: Had she ever done that before?

SUE: No, not really.

THERAPIST: Well, that's really something. If she can be on your side, that's going to help you a lot.

Although these changes did not immediately alleviate the CP Worker's concerns about Kurt going home, she subsequently appeared more able to notice the positive changes undertaken by Kurt and Sue, and more willing to accept the therapist's reports on these changes.

As illustrated in this case of Kurt and Sue, it is important to encourage parents to develop constructive ways to approach and interact with their CP Workers. In general, if parents remain defensive and closed with information, CP Workers are likely to interpret the parents' behavior as indicators of an uncaring attitude or a hostile personality with the potential to abuse. Parents who feel unfairly judged remain angry and resentful, often continuing to interact with their CP Worker in a hostile and rebellious manner, despite having made significant changes in family relationships through the therapy. Because the parents' observable behavior is the CP Worker's only source of direct information about the parents' "changes," it is necessary to help parents adopt a more purposeful and constructive stance in relation to their CP Worker. When this cannot be done through coaching, the therapist can arrange a meeting between the parents and the CP Worker.

Joint Meetings between Parents and CP Workers

There are a number of situations in which it is useful to have joint meetings with CP Workers and parents. These include (1) when parents deny or minimize the extent of the abuse, (2) when parents have difficulty in changing a negative pattern of interaction with the CP Worker, or (3) in order to minimize conflict and develop some common purpose between the parents and CP Worker. Joint meetings should only occur sometime after the "initial meeting," as described in Chapter 4.

When Parents Appear to Deny or Minimize the Abuse

In some cases, the story parents give to the therapist during the initial meeting does not appear to fit with the degree of intervention that has occurred. For example, a single-parent mother said that the Department had removed her infant because she was not coping following a caesarean birth. She reported that she had been too incapacitated to get up and feed the baby at night. We were puzzled that, under such circumstances, her child would be made a permanent ward. When the therapist contacted the CP Worker, the CP Worker said that the mother had been observed hitting the month-old infant. Consequently, the Department was very concerned about the mother having unsupervised access with the child again.

Faced with such discrepant accounts, therapists are in the difficult position of having information that the parent has not disclosed to them. Simply reporting back to the parents the content of the discussion with the CP Worker risks being perceived as taking the CP Worker's side. In these circumstances, it may be necessary to arrange a meeting, during which the CP Worker repeats the story that was previously revealed to the therapist. When suspecting that the parent is not "telling the whole story," it is often useful to foreshadow the possibility of a meeting when the therapist first discusses with the parents the idea of telephoning the CP Worker.

Because CP Workers are sometimes reluctant to tell their full story in front of parents, they can be prepared for the meeting by explaining to them the importance of certain information being revealed in its entirety in front of the parents. When the parents and CP Worker are brought together, it is then possible to explore the situation without appearing to confront the parents directly. Meeting with the CP Worker also allows the parents to present their position and clarify any misunderstandings.

When Parents Appear Unable to Adopt a Strategic Position

Meetings are useful when parents are unable to shift an escalating conflict between themselves and the CP Worker. In the previous example of Kurt and Sue, both quickly caught on to the notion of "catch-22," seeing the situation with some humor. In the example that follows, the parents had been unable to reverse their negative stance towards the CP Worker. They appeared overwhelmed and confused about the policies and practices of the Department, and presented a united front to the CP Worker.

To Develop a Common Purpose between the CP Worker and Parents

A final reason for bringing the parents and the CP Worker together is to help them establish a common purpose when the conflict between them is having a destructive effect on the child. In the following case example, the therapist brought together the CP Worker and the parents for two purposes: (1) to deescalate a long-standing conflict between the two parties, and (2) to help them develop a common purpose of protecting Cindy, the daughter, who had been regularly running away from the foster homes in which she was placed.

Cindy, 13, had alleged to her schoolteacher that her father, Brian, had sexually assaulted her. He denied the allegations and Cindy's mother, Beryl, expressed confusion about whom to believe and refused to insist that Brian leave the home. The Department placed Cindy in a foster home. Brian remained in the home, and a condition of bail was that he not see Cindy. Cindy missed her mother desperately and wanted to return home. On several different occasions, the CP Worker tried to persuade Brian to leave the home and Beryl to separate from Brian so that Cindy could return to live with her mother. This had resulted in angry confrontations between the CP Worker and Brian, who steadfastly refused to move or to do anything the CP Worker suggested. The CP Worker arranged for Beryl to have regular access visits with Cindy every Saturday for 3 hours away from the home. Despite this, Cindy's home-sickness drove her to regularly run away from the foster home, trying to find her way home. The Department had placed Cindy in different foster homes and, on one occasion, in a children's detention center in order to detain her, concerned that she would be sexually assaulted as she roamed the streets.

The family was referred to us from another therapist, who had worked with the mother and Cindy unsuccessfully for several months. The therapist portrayed the situation as hopeless and the referral to us as a last resort, given the father's denial and the mother's apparent inability to take a stand. We had several sessions with both parents during which Brian, on the advice of his lawyer, continued to deny the allegations, claiming that the only problem was "the Welfare's" inappropriate intervention. We understood Brian's refusal to move out and allow Cindy to come home as reflecting his fear that such a move would be seen by the Department and the police as an admission of guilt. Because Cindy's behavior of running away from foster homes was placing her at considerable risk, our immediate goal was to address the conflict between the CP Worker and father that prevented Cindy from having adequate access to her mother. The therapist, therefore, called a meeting of the CP Worker and the parents to discuss this issue. The meeting began with Brian and the CP Worker arguing about the truth of the allegations. The therapist interrupted this process and focused on the mutual concern for Cindy:

CP WORKER: Again, we keep coming back to the same thing, the behavior. You seem to keep looking at her behavior in isolation. And her behavior has been, uh, fairly difficult over quite a period of time. The reason people have been giving you such a hard time is because enough research has been done in these matters to suggest that the kid's behavior *is* because of certain things happening to her.

BRIAN: But have you done any investigating into these allegations or not? Like what the police have charged me with?

CP WORKER: I've done what I'm required to do—I've done what I'm required to do when I receive allegations from a child. *All right?*

BRIAN: But *you* are *not* the Welfare. You are the Department of Child Protection. You are a different kind of batch to the Welfare.

CP WORKER: "Department of Child Protection" is the current name for the old Welfare, if you like.

BRIAN: No, but I'll tell you what. The old Welfare, as I remember, they used to work *with* the parents *and* the children to find out what was wrong. But none of this talk about breaking up marriages, split anything up. They tried to pinpoint what went wrong.

CP WORKER: And you don't think that's been done?

BRIAN: No. Not when you want to take the wife and the children away from the home. To me, that is breaking up our marriage.

CP WORKER: I don't particularly want to break up your marriage, and I don't particularly want to take anyone away from anyone. Any suggestions that have been made to your wife about moving out are purely and simply on the basis that *you* wouldn't move out. Cindy's behavior now, and her behavior for a long time, boils down to that what she disclosed hasn't been brought out into the open before, and now it has been brought out into the open==

BRIAN: ==You're going back to when she was 5 years old, are you?

CP WORKER: *(louder)* I don't know, but there are comments on her school record that her behavior was noticeable enough for people to start putting comments on the record that far back.

THERAPIST: Let me just interrupt you here. Probably what we should do is not talk about this particular aspect of the problem. Because it seems to me that since you (*looking at the CP Worker*) have to do your job, and you (*looking at Brian*) are in a particular legal situation, there isn't any way that the two of you could actually come to any agreement about this today.

CP WORKER: No, there isn't.

BRIAN: I wouldn't back down from him.

THERAPIST: Yeah, I think that for this meeting today it would be best to agree that you don't agree about the situation at the moment. But we are all here because we are concerned about Cindy. So the question would be, given that Cindy has this history of settling in to a foster home and then taking off again in every place she's been, what do we think is going to happen in this new situation, and what are we going to do if she decides to take off again?

BRIAN: In my opinion, it seems that no matter where Cindy is based, she settles down for a few days and then she gets it in her head, and off she goes.

THERAPIST: What ideas do you have about why Cindy takes off?

In the discussion that ensued, it became clear that although the access visits provided contact with her mother, Cindy often complained that she missed her brothers, sisters, and the family dog. As a result of this discussion, Brian offered to be away from the house for 6 hours every Saturday, so that Cindy could come home during that time. The CP Worker accepted this proposal. As the meeting concluded, it was evident that the interaction between Brian and the CP Worker had changed.

BRIAN: Well, I'll tell you what. I reckon that we should of had this a long time ago. We might have got somewhere (*leaning forward and looking at the CP Worker*). Today we've achieved more out it than what we have in the last 2 years, more or less. With the three of us just sitting down with you (the therapist) and having a general discussion on it.

THERAPIST: You feel like you understand his point of view a bit better?

BRIAN: Yes.

CP WORKER: Yes, that's good. I agree.

In subsequent weeks, Cindy's runaways decreased, and Brian's entrenched negative position toward the CP Worker shifted such that he agreed to move out for the entire weekend.

In this, as in other cases considered "hopeless" by professionals, significant, even if limited, changes are possible when the relationship between the CP Worker and parents is addressed.

REPORTING BACK TO THE DEPARTMENT

Parents frequently believe that reports from the therapist to the Department or Courts are indicative of a therapist–CP Worker coalition. To change this perception, and to minimize the experience of betrayal that often results from such reports, traditional reports can be replaced with letters written directly to the parents. Letters are presented and discussed during a therapy session and address the objectives that have been outlined in the initial discussion with the CP Worker.

"Reports" written in the form of letters can have therapeutic impact. By summarizing the therapy and the changes made or yet to be made, the letter can further the parents' motivation toward constructive change. By commenting on and publicly stating the strengths of family members, letters can generate hope, build family members' self-esteem, and increase the positive regard of other professionals for family members. Letters can also provide leverage for change, a subject addressed in the next chapter. Even in those cases where parents are non-English-speaking or illiterate, the letters can be read to family members by the therapist or through the therapist's interpreter.

The following letter was given to Sue and Kurt prior to their return to Court. They gave one copy to their own lawyer and another to their CP Worker. This letter had many purposes: It was feedback to the CP Worker and Court about the couple's progress; it was an intervention that provided positive reinforcement and a public statement of the parents' strengths; and it was also a way to introduce to the CP Worker and Court (via Kurt and Sue) what we saw as the necessary next steps.

Dear Sue and Kurt,

This letter is to summarize our contact to date. Over the last 2 months, I have had 10 sessions with you: four with the two of you, four with you and Andy and Jessica, and one with each of you alone. You have attended every session, always been on time, and participated fully and openly both in the session and with tasks I asked you to undertake between sessions. It has been apparent to me that you both are very committed to each other and concerned about preserving your relationship as partners and as parents.

Over this time, I have come to understand how it was that Kurt hurt the children:

1. Kurt had little experience with children and failed to appreciate just how vulnerable a young child is.

2. Lack of support and validation for your relationship from your own families. This was the result of a family conflict not of your making.

3. Lack of inclusion of Kurt as a parent with Andy and Jessica. Prior to meeting Kurt, Sue had relied on her mother to help raise Andy. When Kurt became involved, there was little room for him as a parent to Andy or, later, to Jessica. This left Kurt feeling excluded and unimportant.

Over the last few months there have been several significant changes. First, Sue's parents have become more supportive of your relationship and of Kurt as a father to Jessica and stepfather to Andy. Second, Sue now sees Kurt as a coparent and discusses decisions regarding the children with him. Both of you have become more open in dealing with your differences and difficulties as parents. Third, Kurt has developed a separate relationship with Andy and Jessica, and no longer sees them as simply taking time away from Sue and himself.

I have been very impressed with how both of you handle Andy and Jessica—in a very gentle and caring manner that is firm and with limits, without relying on physical punishment. You have told me about your desire to learn more about parenting, and Kurt has, himself, sought out resources in the community and signed up for a parenting class to begin later this year. My greatest concern at this stage is that you, Kurt, need to have more opportunities to be a father with Jessica and Andy and a coparent with Sue. I believe that in these 3 months we have addressed many of the issues that we can deal with until the two of you are actually living together. My suggestion to you is that you seek permission to live together again. We can work out a way in which this can be done in a progressive manner, allowing you to work out difficulties as they arise.

Yours sincerely,

Laurie MacKinnon,
Family Therapist.

Once Kurt and Sue delivered a copy of the letter to the Department, we again sought their permission to speak with the CP Worker. The conditions under which the CP Worker would agree to the possibility of the parents reuniting needed to be discussed. During this telephone call, the CP Worker expressed her concerns about the couple reuniting too quickly. We agreed with her and proposed to organize a graduated plan with the parents. This was done in a subsequent interview with Sue and Kurt, who then took a copy of the following letter to the CP Worker. Subsequently, the letters were presented in court by both the CP Worker and the parents' lawyer. The judge agreed to the plan.

Dear Sue and Kurt,

This letter is to summarize our discussions on July 3rd. The following were the ideas you proposed to me about how to reunite in a way that would assure the Department of the safety of Jessica and Andy and provide you with optimum support during this transition phase.

First, this presumes that custody will be restored to Sue.

Week 1. (the first week after the Court) During this week, the four of you will have outings as a family on a few occasions. This means that Kurt, you will pick up Sue and the children from Sue's parents and bring them back to her parent's house the same day. You suggested outings such as going to the park for picnics.

Week 2. During this week, the visits proposed during Week 1 will continue and, in addition, on Thursday afternoon you, Kurt, will pick up Sue and the children to stay with you overnight and return them to Sue's parent's place on Friday afternoon. You suggested that I telephone you sometime that evening to discuss how things are going.

Week 3. During this week, the visit will be extended from Thursday night to Saturday evening, during which time you would like me to telephone you to discuss how things are going.

Week 4. During this week, in addition to the weekday visits, you will be together Thursday night to Saturday evening, and I will not telephone.

Week 5. Provided all has gone well in the previous week, during this week, you will move into your flat together.

During each of the above weeks and over the next month, you will continue to meet with me weekly to discuss the stresses and differences of opinions that arise through these various experiences. In this way you will have an opportunity for weekly support and a place to discuss problems. Both of you also will be attending parenting classes, beginning in April and continuing on a weekly basis.

You have both commented to me on your plans should the stress during any of these times become excessive: Kurt, you said that should it become difficult, you will take time out and separate yourself temporarily from Sue and the children. You will also telephone me to discuss the problem. If at any time you become concerned, Sue, you said that you will telephone me to discuss the problem, as well as bring the issue to the next therapy session. You both understand and are in agreement with the continuing supervision by the CP Worker from the Department.

I would suggest that you forward a copy of this letter to your CP Worker and one to your lawyer so that they may understand your proposal.

Yours sincerely,

Laurie MacKinnon,
Family Therapist

As Sue and Kurt proceeded with this plan, they began to present more issues in therapy about their relationship and uncertainty about taking the final step of living together. They openly conflicted about the expectations they had of each other as marital partners. Kurt complained that Sue expected him to be a traditional husband who provided for her in the middle-class manner to which she had become accustomed in her own family. He said he resented the expectations and felt trapped and helpless. He also felt that Sue's parents were reluctant to let him become a father to Andy. Sue, despite previous denials to the therapist, revealed that Kurt had, on one occasion, hit her during an argument. Kurt initially complained that he "couldn't help it," and that she had "provoked" him to the point that he had been justified in hitting her. Over the next several sessions, however, Kurt took responsibility for this violence and his abuse of the children, and Sue felt less concerned that it would happen again. Nevertheless, as a result of this focus, the couple decided to postpone living together for another few months.

A further complication arose in that even though at this point she was agreeable to their living together, the CP Worker was reluctant to permit Kurt to be alone with the children. The fact that Kurt spent very little time with them, however, was increasingly problematic: Kurt felt on the periphery of the mother–child relationships, and the children consistently preferred their mother to their father. We further negotiated with the CP Worker, and Sue and Kurt proposed another plan in which, over a 5-week period, Kurt would gradually have increasing time alone with each of the children. When the couple presented this next letter to the CP Worker, she agreed to their plan. Some weeks later, the relationship between Kurt and each of the children seemed considerably closer. Kurt said that he now experienced his relationship with Jessica as quite separate from any of the issues between himself and Sue. He also felt he had a secure place with Andy. The couple resumed living together 1 year after therapy had commenced.

Over the course of this therapy, a total of seven letters were sent to the couple, all of which they passed on to both the CP Worker and their lawyer. The positive tone and supportive quality of the letters was unproblematic. It genuinely reflected our perceptions of the couple's progress. There are, however, other situations in which a wholly positive letter cannot honestly be written about a family's progress. In some cases, the situation that led to the abuse in the first place has not changed, the effects of the abuse have not been adequately addressed, or family members have not made the changes the therapist believes are necessary for the child's safety. Even in these situations, it is often possible to write letters to the family rather than report directly to the Department. It is in the parents' interest to pass on all letters to the CP Worker, even those not wholly positive, because without such letters, the parents have no evidence that they have participated in therapy or made any progress at all. These letters must be optimistic but honest and designed to encourage parents to take the next steps. In the case of Sandra and Barry, we found ourselves in such a position.

Sandra, 24, had been living with Barry, 25, for the past year. Sandra had a son, Sam, 7, and a daughter, 4, from a previous relationship. The CP Worker referred the family to us 5 weeks before they were due to return to the Children's Court. The parents had seen a previous therapist who, according to the CP Worker, determined that they were "resistant" and "unable to change." When the first therapist declined to go further with the case, the CP Worker referred them to our center. The CP Worker reported that the stepfather had brutally beaten the son by hand and strap, and that the boy's maternal aunt had noticed bruising on the boy over a period of months. He commented that Sandra had said that "the more the Welfare intervenes, the greater the problem," and he believed that "in a sense, she is right. The more pressure she feels, the worse she is to Sam."

In the "initial meeting" with the family, Barry and Sandra described Sam as having "a negative attitude" toward Barry, evidenced by his refusal to follow through with Barry's instructions when Sandra was at work. Barry claimed that he had "belted" his stepson as a disciplinary measure after Sam had created a scene, when Barry picked him up from school, by refusing to go home with him. The couple described having been "dobbed in" by the maternal aunt, who suspected that Barry was hitting Sam. In response, the parents angrily terminated contact with Sandra's family.

In a telephone call to the CP Worker, we were able to elicit behavioral objectives. The CP Worker explained that he would be reassured and could disengage from the family if the following conditions were present. These conditions, however, he explained, could only apply to Sandra, as Barry was not a legal guardian:

1. Sam was attending school regularly.
2. The school said Sam was doing well.
3. Sandra acknowledged that there was a problem and that "beatings are not OK."
4. Sandra demonstrated other ways of handling the children's behavioral problems. All hitting must stop.
5. Sandra demonstrated that she can deal with emotional issues by talking to the children.
6. Sandra demonstrated willingness to accept court orders for supervision by the Department, counseling, and community-health-nurse access to Sam.

The therapist wrote to the CP Worker summarizing these conditions and the telephone call. A copy of this letter was made available to the parents in the next session, and we discussed ways of working on these conditions as our objectives. The parents seemed relieved to have found some way of getting the CP Worker "off their backs."

The children's court was to determine whether Sam should remain with his mother or be placed in permanent care. By the fifth week, when the family was to return to court, they had achieved all of the objectives that the CP Worker had initially outlined, and relationships within the family had improved considerably. Nevertheless, we remained concerned that Sandra had never forgiven her sister for notifying and had subsequently cut off contact with her mother and sisters, leaving her isolated in a relationship with Barry. We also believed that Sam had suffered over the last few months from the loss of contact with his grandmother, aunts, and cousins. Sandra and Barry, however, were unwilling to reconsider any type of contact with Sandra's family, saying that they would never forgive them.

In the letter to Sandra that we subsequently took to the CP Worker and to her own lawyer, we outlined the many positive changes the couple had made in their relationship with Sam. We also acknowledged, however, that the final step of healing the relationship with Sandra's family had not occurred. Knowing how much the couple resented being ordered to therapy in the first place and were looking forward to the day when they did not have to attend, we attempted to motivate Sandra to take the step of reuniting with the family, with the promise of no further therapy. The following letter was given to Sandra prior to the court appearance.

Dear Sandra,

This is the letter you requested to summarize our contact in therapy to date.

As of today, I have had six sessions with your family. This included one with you and Sam alone, one with you and Barry alone, and four with the three of you. After our initial session, I telephoned the CP Worker and asked him to specify what he saw as suitable goals for therapy. We have subsequently been addressing these objectives. Objectives 1 and 2 had already been achieved prior to my contact with you.

Objective No. 3. In our last session, both you and Barry talked with Sam about the beating, acknowledging that beating is wrong. You both apologized to Sam and assured him that this form of discipline would not be used again. In this session, we also discussed alternative ways of handling Sam's behavior should further discipline be needed.

Objectives Nos. 4 and 5. Following our third session, you and Barry began experimenting with other ways of interacting with Sam, including talking with him to ease his fears, involving him in more activities with you and Barry, and talking more with him about things he has done at school and throughout the day. You have also reported a change in Sam: He appears to initiate affectionate contact more frequently and has responded to your reassurance that you will remain a family. He appears to be spontaneously role modeling after Barry and looking to him as a father. You have made a commitment to not using hitting as a form of discipline.

Objective No. 6. Your willingness to accept the court orders will be apparent when you return to court next Tuesday.

Initially, it was difficult for me to make an accurate assessment of your family, because Sam's association with professionals and the meaning they have for him in terms of being removed from the family inhibit him in the session. However, in our last meeting together, Sam was much more open, spontaneous, and responsive to both you and Barry. This seemed to be a result of you reassuring him that I was attempting to help the family. In this session, it appeared to me that he was responsive to both you and Barry, and did not appear afraid. This was in sharp contrast to our first session.

Given your reluctance to continue with therapy, I would suggest that therapy is not indicated at the present time. However, I am concerned that the effects of intervention have been such that you and Sam have become further alienated from your family. For your family to fully recover from the crisis you have been through, I see it as necessary that the issues in this area be resolved so that Sam may resume a loving relationship with his grandmother, aunts, and cousins. It may not be necessary for you to resume your relationship with your sister for this to occur. I would suggest to you that you ask that you be allowed to work out this problematic area yourself and only use counseling if you are not successful in doing so.

Yours sincerely,

Laurie MacKinnon,
Family Therapist

Although therapy then ended, within a few weeks the CP Worker telephoned to tell the therapist that, on her own accord, Sandra had initiated contact with the grandmother and arranged for Sam and his sister to see their aunts and cousins.

In the cases presented thus far, the CP Worker honored the "contract" the therapist had so painstakingly obtained when the family was first referred. There are, however, situations in which this does not happen. Even well intentioned CP Workers are sometimes overruled by a superior or replaced by another CP Worker who sees the situation differently. The Department may refuse to return the child or allow greater access despite, from the therapist's point of view, the parents having made significant and necessary changes. When this happens in the early or middle stages of therapy, the therapist can take the opportunity to renegotiate the objectives. When the Department's change of position occurs, however, as therapy is concluding, options are fewer.

One option is to request a meeting with the CP Worker and his or her supervisor, explore their concerns, and determine if another stage of therapy with further objectives would address their concerns. Such meetings are not always helpful, however. Supervisors often hold similar opinions and may form a united front with the CP Worker. Arguing with the CP Worker or supervisor is usually unhelpful, as it elicits further defensiveness and determination to be right.

Because these cases usually involve the courts, the courts are the final arbitrator between the parents and the Department. For this reason, it is very important to ensure that parents have separate legal representation in the Children's Court. Unaware of their rights, many parents would otherwise rely solely on the CP Worker's representations to the Court. When we perceive significant positive changes in parents and believe that they are being unfairly treated by the Department not honoring their "contract," we cease negotiating with the Department. Instead, we support parents in having their perspective on the matter heard in the Children's Court and assist them in obtaining legal representation. Although we encourage parents to deal directly with their own lawyers, we are also willing to speak at length with them. We clarify to the parents the importance of their delivering our "letters" to *both* their lawyer and to the CP Worker, rather than relying on the CP Worker to present our "reports" to the Court.

In some work settings, therapists fear that if they encourage parents to use the courts in this way, the Department will begin to see their service negatively and stop referring clients. This is particularly problematic when the Department directly or indirectly funds the therapy or the center. This may indicate a true conflict of interest. If, however, the therapist has handled the cases as outlined in this approach, only a small minority should ever reach a stalemate that must be resolved in court. In the majority of cases, the therapist's service will be a significant improvement on how cases are normally handled, and the CP Worker will feel respected and understood.

CONCLUSION

This chapter has addressed the question of how therapists can position themselves in relation to child protection professionals in cases involving allegations of child abuse. The approach described is one in which the therapist is positioned as a power broker—advocating, negotiating, and mediating between child protection professionals and parents to create a context for therapy that is workable. The therapist advocates on the parents' behalf to minimize authoritarian practices and oppression by professionals, and in order to create hope that therapy might assist the parents in reaching goals as defined by them. Through this process, parents begin to trust the therapist and become more willing to use therapy for intrafamilial issues. The therapist also supports CP Workers in carrying out their responsibilities for ensuring the child's safety by clarifying the specific changes that parents must make. For both CP Workers and parents, the therapist is a negotiator and mediator assisting them to develop relationships that are less authoritarian, less adversarial, and more constructive. The focus of therapy in child-at-risk situations must be directed as much to the relationship between the therapist and CP Worker and the CP Worker and family as it is, ultimately, to the relationship between family members. Therapy fails when therapists who are eager to "do therapy" attempt to deal with intrafamilial issues long before these external issues are resolved.

In the foregoing discussion, we have positioned ourselves as therapists able to take the side of parents in managing a bewildering and complex system that confronts them. The complication of child-at-risk cases, however, is that, as therapists, we cannot simply be advocates for the parents. When a child may be suffering or is in some way at risk, we must be able to also position ourselves in such a way that the parents are interested and motivated to make changes in their own family relationships. As a power broker, the therapist cannot leave this element to chance but must clearly conceptualize and plan the leverage for change available in each situation.

〰

Raising the Stakes in Child-at-Risk Cases: Eliciting and Maintaining Parents' Motivation

THE issue most frequently raised by therapists concerning child-at-risk cases is that parents in these families are extremely resistant to treatment. The manifestation of this resistance boils down to the fact that such clients fail to keep appointments, drop out prematurely, refuse to acknowledge any problems, are closed with information, are often unwilling to follow therapists' directives, and generally appear unmotivated and uninterested. In the previous two chapters, we have outlined ways of beginning therapy in order to create an alliance with parents and help them deal constructively with CP Workers. This chapter addresses how therapists can further construct therapeutic leverage in order to elicit and maintain parents' motivation throughout the course of therapy.

In our work, we sought to minimize both situations where we had to report to the Department and the frequency with which parents terminated therapy following notification to the Department. We also aimed to increase and maintain the motivation of clients. Our overall aim was to develop strategies for effecting at least small changes in the multitude of otherwise "hopeless" situations and "catch 22s" that so often confront therapists dealing with child-at-risk cases.

AN APPROACH TO ELICITING AND MAINTAINING CLIENT MOTIVATION

Because the very fact of the family being in therapy may indicate to police and CP Workers that they need no longer concern themselves with the case, conducting therapy with abusive parents entails certain risks. Therapy may camouflage dangerous situations and increase the likelihood of future abuse going undetected. It is important, therefore, to assess the risk to the child involved in undertaking therapy in each particular situation and to determine whether and how to notify, and the extent of leverage required to proceed safely.

Proceeding Cautiously

Five factors must be considered in judging whether therapy can be safely undertaken.

The Abuser's Access to the Child

Extreme care must be taken when the abuser is still living with, or has unsupervised access to, the child. When a parent who has been abusive is still living with the family, the age of the abused child and the age of other children in the home must be considered. Young children are more vulnerable, will be remaining at home longer, and are less able to seek allies outside the family.

The Type, Extent, and Duration of Abuse

"Abuse" can refer to many different types of behaviors, situations, and degrees of risk. A single occurrence of physical abuse during a time of stress for which the parent feels remorse is quite different from routine bashing justified as discipline. Because of its greater invisibility, greater secrecy, and tendency to reoccur, sexual abuse poses particular risks. Men who sexually assault often describe their behavior as a compulsive and repetitive act. The cessation of the assault in such cases is often temporary, either reoccurring with the same child at a later date or with another child. Victims of sexual assault report that it may reoccur episodically over several years and often involves many children of both genders within a family during different time periods. Short-term therapy with little follow-up in such cases is unlikely to prevent reoccurrence. Therapy should not be undertaken while the perpetrator is still living under the same roof as a young child who has been sexually assaulted.

In any child-at-risk case, it is important to provide individual sessions along with whole family sessions in order to understand the type, extent, and duration of abuse. It is otherwise easy to be very much misled as to the extent and severity of abuse. In the initial interview with a family who requested help for a "communication" problem, for example, the father revealed that he had "touched" his daughter 1 year ago at a time when his marriage was under considerable stress. He left us with the impression that he had fondled his daughter on one or two occasions, an impression his daughter appeared to confirm. It was only when the daughter was interviewed alone that she described how her father had had sexual intercourse with her three to four times a week over a period of 1 year.

The Parents' Attitudes and Responses

Both the abusive and nonabusive parents' attitudes to the abuse and, in cases of sexual assault, their response to the child's disclosure should be considered. The nonabusive parent may believe, support, and be willing to protect the child. The abuser may admit the abuse, feel guilt, remorse, and a desire to change or, alternatively, deny the abuse or appear to feel justified and unrepentant.

When an abusive or nonabusive parent denies the abuse, it is useful to attempt to understand the context of this denial. Some alleged abusers, for example, find their own behavior so abhorrent that they cannot admit it and may fear the loss of their spouse or family and the social and legal consequences of exposure. Nonabusive parents sometimes fear the relationship consequences of acknowledging the abuse or, estranged from their child, view the allegations as manipulative.

Substance Abuse by the Parents

Care must be taken in proceeding with therapy if one or both parents are significantly affected by the use of alcohol or drugs. Although the parents may express concern and positive intent, they may be unable to follow through with behavioral change unless and until there is a change in the abuse of these substances.

Consideration of Other Options

Finally, before undertaking a form of therapy that can have the effect of solidifying a marriage or maintaining the family unit, it is essential that family members are informed about the options available to them. If, for example, parents request family therapy after the father has been violent or sexually abusive to any of the children, it is important to explore in individual sessions with the mother and young person the extent of violence and intimidation, their options concerning separation, and their choices concerning treating the issue as a criminal matter.[1] If the abused young person and the nonabusive parent are of the view that the situation should be treated as a criminal matter, then the therapist can assist them in proceeding in that direction. If, however, they do not, then the therapist is left to consider whether he or she is obligated to notify and, if so, how either to avoid an unnecessary notification or to notify in a constructive manner.

Avoiding Unnecessary Notifications

When therapists are apparently obligated to report the family to the Department but are of the opinion that the child is no longer at risk and that a notification would not be useful, it may be possible to contact the Department unofficially prior to officially reporting the case. Without initially identifying the family, an inquiry can be made about the requirements for reporting given the particular family's circumstances. In the case examples that follow, we believed we were obligated to report but saw little value in doing so. By contacting the Department and having a preliminary discussion, as described, arrangements were made that allowed us to fulfill our legal obligation while still maintaining positive engagement with the clients.

CASE EXAMPLE 1

Don Anderson sexually assaulted his 15-year-old daughter, Sarah, on five occasions over a 1-month period. While his wife had been at work, Don had entered his daughter's room and touched her genitals while she was sleeping. Upset and afraid, Sarah disclosed to her mother after the last incident, when her mother, Jeanine, confronted her husband and insisted that he leave the home. Two months later, the couple sought "marriage counseling."

We believed that we were legally required to notify the sexual abuse of a minor. However, we feared jeopardizing the parents' engagement in therapy and saw little to gain by notifying, given that the daughter was not at risk. We did not want charges brought against her father, who was living away from home, and the mother remained supportive and protective of the daughter.

Without disclosing the family's identity, the therapist telephoned the Department's office and described the family's circumstances to the CP

---

[1]In all of the cases described in this chapter, this step was taken before we proceeded any further with therapy for the family.

Worker on intake. The CP Worker concluded that given the particular circumstances, nothing could be gained by notification. The therapist recorded the details of this conversation in the case file and did not make a formal report to the Department.

CASE EXAMPLE 2

Eric Stevens, 14, was sexually assaulted by his father on one occasion several years ago. His parents subsequently divorced, and he has had only occasional contact with his father since. When, in the course of family therapy, he disclosed the incident, he expressed concern at the possibility of the therapist notifying and charges being brought against his father.

Without identifying the client, the therapist telephoned the Department and discussed the situation with the CP Worker on intake. The CP Worker determined that the therapist need not notify immediately but must do so at some stage. The therapist continued to work with the mother and son, and some months later the son indicated his readiness to speak with the CP Worker.

In both these situations, the young person was no longer at risk of abuse, and there was little to gain from the notification. Notification was either avoided or its impact was minimized while the therapist remained within legal and policy guidelines. Given the particularities of each situation and the frequency with which policies change and differ from state to state, it is not possible to prescribe here precisely when therapists should or should not notify. Taking each situation on an individual basis and contacting the Department for a discussion prior to notification are the best options for therapists in ambiguous situations.

Notifying Constructively

Whether faced with reporting the family to the Department because of a requirement to do so, or because it appears necessary for the safety of the child to do so, the notification ought to be conceptualized as *part of* rather than *outside of* the therapy process. By anticipating the effects of notifying and the subsequent investigation, it is possible to take a number of steps to lessen the parents' sense of betrayal and to facilitate the parents' cooperation with the process.

Obtain Information from the Department

When contacting the Department to clarify whether a particular case must be notified, further information may be obtained regarding the

Department's practices and procedures, and how these might be negotiated. This can be done by asking hypothetical questions of the CP Worker concerning the notification and investigation of this case. For example, some of the following questions might be asked:

> "If my report to the Department is accepted as a notification, what will be the likely course of events?"
> "If I must report, when must it occur?"
> "Are there alternative ways of proceeding with the investigation following notification, for example, by the CP Worker interviewing the parent at my office or with me being present with the parent at their home during the interview?"

Provide Support and Choices

Before making a notification, it is advisable in most cases that the parents be told what is going to happen and why notification is necessary. During this discussion, the parents' motivation in initiating therapy is recognized and acknowledged, concern is expressed for both parents and children, and the parents are assured of the therapist's commitment to stand by them during any subsequent investigation.

The options available concerning how and by whom the notification will be made, and the implications of each option are then openly discussed. For example, the parents may be able to choose whether the therapist or they themselves will make the notification, and where and with whom the parents' initial meeting with the CP Worker will take place. Options include inviting the CP Worker to the next therapy session, arranging for the therapist to be with the family at their home during the investigation, or arranging for the parents to visit an office of the Department themselves.

In discussing these options, it is useful to keep in mind that if the parents notify themselves, the Department is likely to be less concerned than if the notification is made from someone outside the family. When the therapist is seeking to soften the Department's involvement, the parents should be encouraged to notify themselves. However, there are situations in which the therapist and/or the parents desire a more active intervention from the Department. In those cases, the notification should be made by the therapist or someone else outside the family.

One exception to the principle of providing choices involves situations of sexual assault. If the abuse has not been acknowledged by the parents, and if it is likely that it will be denied by the perpetrator, advance notice of the Department's investigation should not be provided. In such a case, notice may allow the parents to close ranks and silence the child before he or she has been interviewed by the Department.

Prepare the Parents for the Investigation

Before the parents' meeting with the Department, therapists can prepare the parents by providing as much detailed information as possible concerning the Department's purposes and procedures, and the likely outcome of the investigation. If the Department's involvement might assist the parents in some way, the therapist can remain positive about the outcome of the notification without raising false hopes. Although referral to the Department may assist the family in obtaining emergency housing, for example, a promise of this type risks the parents becoming disillusioned and angry if it is not fulfilled.

By explaining the wide variation in personal styles of CP Workers, it is possible to explore with the parents how to handle an encounter with an unfriendly or aggressive CP Worker. In some cases, parents can be coached to respond in a more cooperative manner to a situation that would otherwise elicit their defensiveness. Following the investigation, and preferably within 1 or 2 days, it is important to meet with the family to debrief the experience, allowing family members to ventilate any anger and frustration within a supportive context.

CASE EXAMPLE 3

Peter Lambert, 36, had intercourse with his 14-year-old daughter, Lara, over a period of 1 year. He ceased the assaults when Lara disclosed to her mother. Two months later, fearing that his wife would leave him, Peter initiated family therapy and confided to the therapist that he had "touched" Lara.

In meeting with family members individually, the extent of the abuse was revealed. The therapist was legally required to notify and was also concerned about undertaking therapy while Peter was still living in the home with this daughter and two younger sisters. At the same time, the therapist was also concerned about the effect that notification would have on Peter's motivation to continue in therapy. Meeting separately with Peter and his wife, she explained to them her concerns for the children and her obligation to report. She outlined the various ways in which notification could take place. Through this discussion, Peter chose to report his behavior directly to the Department himself. The next day, he visited a Department office, where he disclosed his actions to the CP Worker on intake and asked for the Department's help.

After interviewing Lara, the CP Worker concluded that the situation would not be reported to the police so long as Peter moved out of the family home and continued in therapy. Peter moved out the following day and remained committed to therapy.

CASE EXAMPLE 4

Over a 3-month period, Daniel Kopel sexually assaulted his 13-year-old stepdaughter, Alice, by fondling her and exposing himself on three occasions. Alice disclosed to her mother, Marion, who confronted Daniel and threatened to leave unless he agreed to marital therapy. On the advice of a family friend who had apparently reassured the couple that notification to the Department or the police was not necessary, the Kopels sought marital therapy.

When informed during the first session that the therapist believed she was legally required to notify, the parents were upset and dismayed. The couple chose the option of the CP Worker being invited to a therapy session. The therapist prepared them for the meeting with the CP Worker by coaching them to remain open and nondefensive in the face of aggressive questioning. The CP Worker attended the next session, and the parents appeared to remain calm and cooperative during the investigation. When the therapist met with them afterwards, however, and elicited their feelings about the interview, they described the CP Worker as judgmental and dogmatic. They said they were angry and upset both with the CP Worker and the therapist. The therapist empathized with their experience and validated their perception of the harshness of the CP Worker's manner. She also acknowledged their anger at her for involving the Department and predicted that it would take them some time before they could trust her again.

When, as in the previous case example, parents experience the notification and subsequent investigation as negative, they may terminate therapy despite the therapist's best efforts to keep them engaged. In such situations, it is essential to have in place some form of leverage that will ensure that the parents remain in therapy.

Maintaining Parents' Motivation through Therapeutic Leverage

The presence of factors that increase parents' interest and commitment to therapy creates *therapeutic leverage*. Leverage may be of three types: that which ensures the safety of family members while therapy is being conducted, that which ensures that parents regularly attend therapy, and that which motivates parents to remain open and interested in examining and changing attitudes, behavior, and relationships. Leverage may be inherent within particular situations or may be elicited and constructed by the therapist. In the presence of therapeutic leverage, therapy with child-at-risk cases becomes possible.

Leverage can be constructed or elicited when the therapist has some influence over a situation, event, or relationship that is valued by the parent. In looking for potential avenues of leverage, consider what the parent is wishing to avoid (such as a child being removed from the home), or what the parent desires to have (such as a father wanting to return home, a parent wanting a closer relationship with a spouse or child). Because the form of available leverage often changes over the course of therapy, it is important to remain constantly aware of the type of leverage being employed and to gauge its effectiveness. Child-at-risk cases bog down and become risky when no replacement is sought for the leverage that was initially available. There are a number of alternative forms of leverage available to therapists.

The Threat to Notify

In some cases, the only initial form of leverage available is the threat to notify the Department or the police. Although such a form of leverage may be effective to some extent, it also positions the therapist negatively and should be replaced as soon as possible by leverage that positions the therapist as helpful to the parents in meeting their goals.

CASE EXAMPLE 5

Return to the situation of Don Anderson (Case Example 1), who had sexually assaulted his 15-year-old daughter. In this case, the CP Worker had indicated that notification was not necessary, given that the family was in therapy, the father had moved out of the home, and the daughter was no longer at risk. When the therapist conveyed to the family the CP Worker's position, Don Anderson responded by saying that he would now return home. To this, his wife, Jeanine, remained silent and did not object. The therapist replied that if Don returned home, his daughter would again be at risk, and the therapist would once again be compelled to inform the Department. Stating to Don that it would be at least 6 months before he could return home, she explained that he must make a number of changes before reuniting with them. Consequently, Don agreed to remain living apart and to continue in therapy.

Using Notification to Effect Change

The notification itself may be employed as a form of leverage when parents are encouraged to make changes in order to reduce the negative consequences of the subsequent investigation. By presenting the parents with options prior to the notification, parents can be urged to take actions that will portray their situation in a better light. In cases of sexual assault, for example, it can be predicted to the parents that the Department will take a harsher view of the situation if the father is living with the family and may then explore the option of his voluntarily moving out of the home prior to the notification being made. With the father out of the home, therapy can be conducted with less risk, and leverage may become available in the form of his desire to return home. This was the case, for example, with Daniel Kopel (Case Example 4). Prior to notification, the therapist discussed with Daniel and his wife their options in how the notification could be made. After the therapist foreshadowed the possibility of harsher treatment from the Department should Daniel remain in the home, Daniel chose to move out and rent a flat in a nearby suburb. The therapist also liaised with the CP Worker prior to the Department meeting with the parents to ensure that the Department specified that the police would be informed should Daniel return home or fail to remain in therapy.

Using the Desire to Avoid Punishment

Criminal charges can be used as leverage when parents hope that punishment can be reduced through cooperation in therapy. This form of leverage, however, is only useful while criminal charges are pending and not once the outcome of charges is determined. Although it is sometimes assumed that parents who are motivated to attend therapy by the desire to avoid punishment are insincere in their desire to change, the threat of punishment is a legitimate and sometimes the only initial point of leverage. Once engaged in therapy, other forms of leverage can then be created.

CASE EXAMPLE 6

Arthur Dale, 60, who had exposed himself on one occasion to his daughter's niece, feared that he was facing a jail sentence. He presented to therapy depressed and anxious that his wife would leave him if he went to jail. After the initial meeting with Arthur, the therapist contacted his legal advisers and obtained information regarding the changes Arthur could make that would be recognized at the time of the trial. The therapist developed a secondary form of leverage by meeting alone with Arthur's wife and helping her formulate and present to Arthur a list of conditions that had to be met for her to continue the relationship with him. Experiencing some hope, Arthur attended therapy regularly, examined the reasons for his inappropriate behavior, and made a number of changes both in terms of his sexuality and in relation to his wife. He was able to face the effects of his actions on the child he abused. Experiencing genuine remorse, he apologized to the victim and her family, and attempted to make reparation to his wife. Arthur was sentenced to 3 months in jail, less time than he feared, after which he returned to live with his wife and carry out his work.

Negotiation with the Department to Set Conditions

When families are referred or ordered to therapy by the Department, leverage can be created by negotiating with the CP Worker to set conditions that, once fulfilled, will allow the parents to achieve their desired outcome (such as the Department returning the child to the parents). These conditions must specify changes in family members' behavior that would be evidence that the problem has changed and that the parents are ready for their stated goals. These conditions should be perceived as coming from the Department, not the therapist, and they must be specific and achievable. Further details and case studies involving this form of leverage were reported in the previous two chapters.

Using the Desire for a Good Report

When parents require a positive report to present to the Department, the Children's Court, or the Criminal Court, it is possible to threaten to withhold the report unless further changes are made. This may only be effective, of course, if the parents continue to experience the therapist as caring and supportive.

CASE EXAMPLE 7

Sandra, 24, had been living with Barry, 25, for the past year. Sandra had a son, Sam, 7, and a daughter, 4, from a previous relationship. Barry and Sandra described Sam as having a "negative attitude" toward Barry. Barry claimed that he had "belted" his stepson as a disciplinary measure after Sam had refused to go home with him when Barry had picked him up from school. Angry both at being notified by Sandra's sister and at how the investigation had been handled by the Department, Barry and Sandra resented being ordered to attend therapy. Both, however, made significant changes in therapy and in doing so met many of the conditions the therapist had negotiated with the Department at the time of their referral.

After several weeks of therapy, the parents said that Sam's behavior and the relationship with Barry was significantly improved, and that they saw no need for further therapy. The therapist, however, still perceived Sam as withdrawn and frightened, and was concerned about terminating at this stage. Using the leverage inherent in the parents' desire for a good report to take back to the Children's Court, the therapist told them that although she believed children should be with their parents, to write a letter of support, she would have to have evidence that Sam was no longer at risk. In the session, she said, Sam appeared very frightened.

Countering that Sam did not appear frightened or withdrawn at home, the parents argued that the therapist was misinterpreting Sam's behavior and proposed that Sam acted frightened in the sessions because he was afraid the therapist would again remove him from the family. If this was so, stated the therapist, Sam must have some scars left over from the trauma, whether these were from the belting itself or from the temporary separation that followed the investigation. Both parents agreed that this could be possible, and the therapist discussed with them ways "to help Sam overcome the effects of the trauma."

The parents reassured Sam that they had found nonviolent ways to deal with his misbehavior. On their own accord, Barry and Sandra devised activities and special "talking sessions" with Sam at home. They reassured Sam that he would not be separated from his home and mother again, and that he had nothing to fear from his therapist in this regard. Within two sessions, the therapist no longer perceived Sam as frightened. He appeared to be the affectionate and spontaneous boy the parents described. Barry also appeared to have changed, and he portrayed a softer and gentler manner in interacting with Sam. By the end of therapy, the therapist was reassured that Sam was no longer at risk.

Using Family Members to Create Conditions and Consequences

Leverage may be created by working with key family members in order to create or develop conditions that the abusive parent has to fulfill. The failure to fulfill these conditions would result in consequences the abusive parent would deem undesirable. When the parents have a strong extended-family network, as may be the case with an immigrant family, a therapist who is familiar with their culture may choose to involve influential kin in helping to create leverage.

One of the most powerful consequences is the loss or threatened loss of significant relationships. The woman who has always threatened to leave an abusive husband may be supported in doing so. If she has already left and is considering returning, the therapist may restrain her return, helping her to specify the changes that the husband must make before he can reunite with the family. The therapist can assist the husband to cooperate and accept these conditions by exploring with him his feelings of isolation, the loss of close relationships, and his desire to heal these relationships.

In the following examples, the mother and adolescent children were assisted in identifying behaviors that were isomorphic to the abuse, such as the father's intimidation and autocratic control. These behaviors of the fathers had in both cases maintained the subservient position of the women and, in this sense, left them less able to stand up for and protect their children.

CASE EXAMPLE 8

With the Anderson family (Case Examples 1 and 5), the therapist sought to develop a form of leverage that involved the mother, Jeanine, setting conditions for her husband's return home. The therapist worked intensively in individual sessions with Jeanine and the children, taking them to a point where, in a subsequent session, they confronted Don with a list of conditions for his return. In addition to the condition that he was not to sexually assault his daughter again, they required the following:

1. That he not hit, threaten to hit, or verbally intimidate any family member.
2. That he participate in household chores and maintenance to a degree perceived as fair by Jeanine (both parents worked in paid employment outside of the home).
3. That Jeanine and the children had a say in all decisions that affected the family.
4. That Jeanine had equal say and control over the couple's income and expenditures.

The therapist was thus freed from using the threat of notification as leverage and was consequently able to align with Don in helping him meet these conditions.

CASE EXAMPLE 9

John Orczy sexually assaulted two of his daughters, now aged 16 and 17, intermittently over a period of several years. The assaults ceased when, concerned about his youngest daughter's behavior and wanting help for her, John confessed the situation to his wife, Rita. Although Rita was distraught and overwhelmed with his disclosure, she was determined to remain in the marriage as well as to seek help for her children, herself, and for John.

Because both daughters were over the age of 16, the case was not notifiable to the Department. The youngest daughter had threatened suicide when her father disclosed to her mother, fearing that her father would go to jail. Neither daughter wanted criminal charges laid. Although both parents appeared sincere and motivated in their request for therapy, we anticipated that there would be periods when John's commitment to therapy and to changing his own behavior would wane. We wanted to guard against him "slipping" in his behavior and dropping out of therapy.

John described himself as a small man with a violent temper and related a history of having been neglected and sexually abused as a child. He said he experienced the sexual abuse of his daughters as a compulsive act over which he had little control. His wife and children reported that although John had never actually been physically abusive, they had always lived in fear and intimidation of his threats of violence and his moody nature.

During the early part of therapy, the therapist met with family members separately. During these sessions, she explored with John his fears of losing his wife and children, and convinced him that he needed their help in setting limits for his behavior. In separate interviews, she convinced Rita of the necessity of standing up to John and setting severe consequences for his intimidating behavior or further incidents of abuse. Similarly, in sessions with each of the daughters, the therapist assisted them to set conditions on their father's behavior. In a subsequent family session, the therapist facilitated the encounter between John and Rita, in which he requested these limits and she set them:

JOHN: I want you to be able to trust me. If you're talking to me, I want you to be able to believe me, because I want to tell you how I feel. I want our love to grow. I know that it's shaky at the moment, but I want you to keep on loving me. I will never deceive you or anything, because I love you.

RITA: And you know if you do, it's finished, don't you?

JOHN: I do. Put it this way: I've ruined so many people in my life, even before I met you, good friends that I've deceived, and I don't want to go on ruining any more lives. And I want people to be able to trust me.

THERAPIST: You wanted to ask for Rita's help in terms of keeping you on track.

JOHN: I need some help from you, Rita.

RITA: You know I'm always there. You can talk to me any time about anything.

JOHN: And I don't want you to be afraid of me, either.

RITA: I'm not anymore, actually (*shaking her head*).

JOHN: Because I will never hit you.

RITA: Well, if you do, I'll walk out the door.

JOHN: Well, if I ever hit you or get violent in any way, or in any way threaten the girls, you are to call the police.

RITA: No, I'll go. I'll go, and then I'll call the police. I'll walk out the door. No man will hit me again.

JOHN: I've got violence within me, but I can't really hit anybody unless I go over the boil.

RITA: What if I yelled and screamed back at you? Would you punch me in the face?

JOHN: I probably would have hit you before. I'm that sort of person. Like with workmates, there's always been a fistfight or something.

RITA: But see, now, if you annoy me, I need to be able to argue to correct it, whereas before, I always had to push it inside. Now, I need to be able to have a go at you in anger without being afraid that I'll get belted one. I feel I need that right.

JOHN: Yeah, you've got that right.

RITA: And I have the right to tell you when you're angry that I don't like how you're having a go at the girls.

JOHN: It should be able to be on that level without escalating.

RITA: That's always held me back. And I've always felt resentful that I've never been able to say that I'm angry. I've done it with you, and I've done it with my father. I've never argued back. And now I'm starting to. I had a go at my father the other day when he rang up! I had a go at him, and so he backed off! It was such a shock.

THERAPIST: So you're protecting yourself a bit more now?

RITA: Yes.

THERAPIST: Well I think that's exactly the kind of stance that John needs to hear from you. Like John said, it works as a sort of deterrent, like a crutch, until he can make more changes inside himself.

JOHN: That's right, I don't want to go back.

The therapist asked John to talk to his daughters about what they should do if they ever felt intimidated by him again. He replied that they should "come straight out and tell me" and added that if they remained afraid, they should tell their mother. If, on the other hand, they experienced him acting in a sexualized way, he said, they should go directly to their mother. Both daughters assured him that they would report any incidents or feelings of discomfort to their mother and stated that should John assault anyone ever again, they would both tell their stories to the police and ask for criminal charges to be laid. John said that he "knew the consequences" and that the threat of jail sentence was a deterrent that he needed.

Using Hypothetical Questioning to Create a Shift in Position

The secrecy, guilt, shame, and threat of legal and relationship consequences often fixes the abusive person and others into rigid and unmovable positions on issues that, in the long run, work against all concerned. In such situations, hypothetical questions may allow a person who steadfastly maintains one position to see issues from a different perspective. This shift in perspective is sometimes sufficient for the person to change either his or her position or an aspect of his or her behavior, which, in turn, promotes further changes on the part of others.

The hypothetical ("what if") mode may also be used when allegations of abuse are denied and efforts to confront or deal directly with the alleged abuser have proven unsuccessful. Hypothetical questions may be used to elicit the underlying reasons for the denial (if a person did commit the alleged act, and if he did admit to this act, what did he imagine would be the consequences?) and to explore the context in which the alleged abuse occurred, allowing the therapist to construct a story of the abuse even in the face of the alleged abuser's denial.

Although it is sometimes useful to ask hypothetical questions directly of the alleged abuser, questions addressed to other family members often yield very useful information and may have the impact of unbalancing fixed relationship positions. Acknowledgment of the abuse should not be the goal of hypothetical questioning of this sort, for in pushing a particular view too hard, the therapist is more likely to elicit an undesired response, such as locking the alleged abuser into an even more rigid stance. Family members must experience the therapist as truly maintaining a curious, "what if" position.

CASE EXAMPLE 10

Cindy Hilbert, 13, had alleged to her schoolteacher that her father, Brian, had sexually assaulted her. He denied the allegations, and Cindy's mother, Beryl, expressed confusion about whom to believe and refused to insist that Brian leave the home. The Department placed Cindy in a foster home. Brian remained in the home, and the condition of bail was that he not see Cindy. Cindy missed her mother desperately and wanted to return home. On several different occasions, the CP Worker tried to persuade Brian to leave the home and Beryl to separate from Brian. This had resulted in angry confrontations between the CP Worker and Brian, who steadfastly refused to move or do anything the CP Worker suggested. As a result of the therapist convening a meeting of the parents and CP Worker, Brian agreed to leave the house for 6 hours each Saturday. Although this had improved the situation considerably for Cindy, she still pined to come home each weekend.

In a session with the parents, the therapist explored the question of Brian moving out for the entire weekend so that Cindy, who was now at boarding school, could return to the family home for this period. The topic had been initiated by Beryl telling the CP Worker that she was considering renting a flat so that she could spend the weekends there with Cindy. In the following excerpt, the therapist spoke to the mother in the presence of the father, asking other-oriented hypothetical questions concerning, first, Beryl's idea of getting a flat and, second, the notion of Brian moving out instead:

THERAPIST: If you were to, say, ask Brian to move out into a flat on weekends, instead of you, so that Cindy could go home for the weekend, how do you think he would respond?

BERYL: Oh, no, I could never do that. He would never move out.

THERAPIST: But if you did ask him, how do you think he would respond?

BERYL: He would just get very angry with me for even thinking about it.

THERAPIST: I see. Why do you think that would be? What do you think it would mean to him if you did ask him?

BERYL: He would reckon that I was taking steps to split us up. And that I was keeping him away from the children.

THERAPIST: Would that be what you were intending?

BERYL: No, I don't want to split up. I just want Cindy to be able to be with me for the weekends, and to be with the other children. She really misses her brothers and sisters.

After exploring this issue further, the therapist turned to the father, who had sat quietly throughout the previous interchange, and asked hypothetical questions directly to him.

THERAPIST: Brian, how do you think Beryl is reading you? How do you think you would respond if Beryl asked you to move out on the weekends?

BRIAN: I will move out on the weekends.

THERAPIST: (*puzzled*) You will move out on the weekends?

BRIAN: Yes, I will.

THERAPIST: I see. If you did move out on the weekends, where do you think you would go?

BRIAN: I could probably stay at Pete's place, my mate from work. It's close enough that I can still pick up my son to take him to soccer on Saturday morning.

THERAPIST: If you decided to move out on the weekend, when do you think you would decide to begin doing it?

BRIAN: Next weekend, if it's OK with Pete.

There are several reasons why this interview precipitated such a change. First, by the therapist exploring the possibility with Beryl of getting a flat on weekends, as well as what it would mean to Brian if she asked him to move out instead, Brian was allowed the time to consider his position and given a chance to reconstruct the meaning of moving out. Moving out ceased to be equated with admitting his guilt and conceding to the CP Worker's demands. Second, in keeping with the symmetrical interaction between the couple, and between Brian and the CP Worker, the position Brian finally adopted was one in opposition to that which both the CP Worker and Beryl portrayed of him. Last, as a result of this discussion, Brian could choose to initiate the move rather than feel coerced into it. Despite never admitting the allegations, Brian did move out that weekend and each weekend for the next several months.

CASE EXAMPLE 11

After 1 year of therapy that addressed his sexual assault of his teenage daughter, Gary Doyle revealed to the therapist that 2 years previously, his son, Russell, then 17, was accused of touching a 4-year-old girl who was in his mother's care. The girl disclosed to her parents, a police investigation ensued, and Russell denied the allegations. With too little evidence to lay charges, the police recommended that Russell see an individual therapist. The therapist, however, terminated therapy after a few sessions, stating that he could make no progress, because Russell continued to deny the accusations. Gary and his wife, Judy, both feared that Russell was, in fact, guilty, but faced with his denial, they dropped the issue and had not discussed it again.

In bringing the issue to the current therapy, Gary revealed his own guilt and concern about his son's behavior. He feared that Russell was modeling after himself and may have had unconscious knowledge of his father's sexual assault of Russell's sister. Concerned that he had replicated with Russell his relationship with his own domineering and violent father, he saw Russell as an exceedingly shy, timid, and broken young man.

When Russell, now 19, returned to live with his parents, Gary asked him to attend a few therapy sessions. The first of these sessions had focused on the relationship between father and son. Russell said he perceived his father as very different from his former self, and an initial trust developed between the two. Russell did not know that the therapist knew of the allegations against him, nor that the parents had planned to raise the issue during the following session. In the transcript that follows, hypothetical questioning allowed us to explore and construct a contextual understanding of Russell's behavior and create opportunities for both Russell and his parents to shift from positions in which they had been fixed. The therapist began the session by inquiring about the relationship between Russell and his father since the last session and then asked what they would like to talk about. Judy raised her concern that the issue of the accusations against Russell had never been resolved. As the therapist explored the nature of the allegations, Russell appeared increasingly embarrassed and uncomfortable, his face reddened, and his eyes averted. The following discussion ensued:

THERAPIST: Russell, do you think that your parents now think that you did molest Janie or not?

RUSSELL: I dunno, no idea. I know Dad kinda thinks that I didn't do it. I'm not too sure about Mum.

JUDY: Well, I'm not sure myself. I'm so totally confused, you know? I'm just not sure. But if he has, he can get help, which is the main thing, as long as he's truthful.

THERAPIST: Just let's say hypothetically, I mean, if hypothetically he did do it, what sense would you now make of him doing it?

JUDY: It could have been emotional, like anger, I suppose, rejection, same as Gary. Russell was going through a rather traumatic time. He was trying to get work and he had too much time on his hands, and he was bored. I think at times he was angry with the kids in the house. Little children, you know. He'd come home and there'd be kids everywhere. But, I mean, that was the only way I could earn money to pay the house off. So, could have been from that, I don't know.

At that time, finances were tight. As a laborer, Gary made hardly enough money to support the family. In order to buy their home, Judy had taken children into the home and provided child care. At that time, she was caring for five children.

THERAPIST: What sense would you make of it, Gary?

GARY: Yes, it's true what Judy said, uh, it could be a lot emotional. He might have even seen me with his sister. 'Cause I never know his unconscious. I was a bit worried about some of the books he reads, you know, I mean sort of pornographic. I can't read 'em, because I know what they do to me. But I'm a bit worried lately, what they do to Russell.

THERAPIST: If Russell had done it, and if he wanted to now get some help or talk about it, or whatever, how do you think he thinks you would react?

JUDY: I hope he'd feel that I'd react the same way as I am to his father. I've always loved him. I've loved him all the time, no matter what he did I'd still love him. Even though I got *angry* then. I regret that very much. I think I did of lot of damage. But I'd hope I wouldn't get angry now.

THERAPIST: Do you think that he'd think you'd get angry now?

JUDY: I don't think so, now, because of the way I am with his father.

THERAPIST: (*to Gary*) What do you think he would think you would react like?

GARY: Well, I hope he wouldn't sort of think I would be angry with him, because he'd know the state I'm in and what I've gone through, you know? And, you know, I admitted what I've done. I think, maybe, at the time when I first told him what I had done, he might have thought to himself, "I went through all that, and he was actually doing it, and I wasn't." (*to Russell*) Would that be right?

RUSSELL: Oh, I suppose.

THERAPIST: (*to Russell*) How do you think your parents would react? Do you think they would be more likely to be supportive or more likely to be angry with you?

RUSSELL: I dunno, it's hard to say.

THERAPIST: (*to Russell*) If one was to be supportive, who do you think would be more supportive, your mum or your dad?

RUSSELL: Uh—well, it depends, I suppose.

THERAPIST: If you compare Gary's relationship with his dad, and Russell's relationship with Gary—in terms of the sort of feeling of oppression, how would you compare that?

JUDY: Um, I don't think that between Gary and Russell would be as bad as between him and his dad, because, um, part of the time Gary was an adult and he was trying to be a good father. So at those times when Russell really needed Gary, he's been there for him, whereas Gary's father had never been there really for Gary.

GARY: Couple of times he's helped me out—you know—like real sticky situations, that I've never wanted to go to him, put it that way. So—er—he's never been able to help me, because I've never confided in him.

THERAPIST: (*to Judy*) Do you think, it terms of saying for a young guy, at that time, 17, do you think that Russell would have felt himself to have some sort of influence, power, or whatever in the family, or do you think he would have felt himself to be quite uninfluential, powerless, one down?

JUDY: Yes.

THERAPIST: The second one?

JUDY: Yes.

THERAPIST: And what do you think?

GARY: The same.

THERAPIST: Do you agree with that Russell?

RUSSELL: Um, yeah.

THERAPIST: That was very tough time, for you?

RUSSELL: Yeah, it was—very.

THERAPIST: (*to Russell*) In relation to what would you have felt that way the most—in relation to your dad or your mum, or having the kids in the house, or what sorts of things would make you feel that way the most. The most sort of powerless one down?

RUSSELL: Er—er—Just, er, Dad being sarcastic, things like that.

GARY: I put you down.

THERAPIST: More feeling dictated to?

RUSSELL: Yeah, yeah.

THERAPIST: And could you ever stand up to him, or were you pretty oppressed by him?

RUSSELL: If he was, say, in a bad mood, I couldn't handle it, something like that.

THERAPIST: But you couldn't challenge that? You were just suffering under it?

RUSSELL: That's right.

The therapist's use of hypothetical questioning during this interview allowed the parents to consider how they wanted to respond to Russell and highlighted for Russell his parents' commitment to standing by and helping him. The exploration of why Russell might have abused a child shed light on Russell's life situation, his position within the family, the intimidation he experienced from his father, and the feelings of power-lessness in his own life.

Russell did not admit to the allegations. Following this interview, however, Russell requested several individual sessions in which he dis-cussed his relationship with his father, his desire to develop more egali-tarian relationships than he had seen in his parents' marriage, and his fears in asserting himself with workmates. Over the next year, Gary and Russell developed a closer, warmer relationship, and Russell became more confident and satisfied in his outside relationships.

Whereas in both this, and the previous case example, the outcome of therapy would have been more satisfying had the alleged abusers admitted the allegations and taken responsibility for their behavior, the "catch-22" both men faced in doing so meant that they were unwilling to take this step. Hypothetical questioning in both instances was able to shift individuals from their fixed positions to, in the first case, have the father make a move that was critical to his daughter's happiness, and in the second, allow inroads into a young man reassessing and changing his values and relationships.

CONCLUSION

The family therapy literature has treated the question of coercion into therapy as if it were something negative or outside of the therapeutic process. If, however, we broaden our focus and ask why it is that people at any time subjects themselves to the enforced change and rigorous self-examination of the therapeutic process, we might find that in almost all instances, even where clients appear totally voluntary, there is behind the scenes some form of push or pain that can be understood as therapeutic leverage. This can take the form of fear of losing one's love, job, or of the internal pain associated with grief or loss of self-esteem. What is different in child-at-risk cases is that *it does matter*—indeed, a child's life may be at stake—whether such fear, pain, or promise is great enough to sustain the parents throughout the course of what may be a long and emotionally tumultuous therapy.

In this chapter, we have argued that in child-at-risk cases, the creation of therapeutic leverage cannot be left to chance or circumstance but must be accepted as one of the therapist's primary tasks. Rather than shun this task as "social control" and define it as outside of rather than a part of the therapeutic process, we must embrace the task with creativity and commitment. In doing so, we may become more able both to keep abusive parents in therapy and to create a context within which family members can rewrite the story of the abuse and develop fairer and more equitable relationships.

Rewriting the Story
of Abuse

THE last few chapters have concentrated on the outer ring of relation-ships—the parents and the child protection system, the child protection system and therapy, and the parents and therapists. Developing workable relationships at these outer rings and constructing and maintaining lev-erage is what makes possible a move to what is commonly regarded as "real therapy" with family relationships. Although these phases are often distinct and conducted over separate sessions of therapy, sometimes they are not. As was evident in the case of Kurt and Sue (Chapter 6), when the parents tell their story of intervention during an initial meeting, information about both the incidents of abuse and family relationships is often provided simultaneously. Although the therapist silently registers this information, it may not be attended to until engagement is less tenuous because of the parents' negative experiences associated with the coerced or reluctant referral to therapy. Once clear objectives for therapy are in place, and the parents are more trusting, we enter the next ring of therapy: obtaining the story of abuse and rewriting the family's history of relationships in terms of their experiences of power and powerlessness. When a family is self-referred, rather than referred from the Department, this ring is often entered earlier, often during the first interview.

The genealogical approach, as described in Chapter 4, is on the one hand, a conceptual scheme that allows us to conceptualize the evolution of relationship conflicts over time and their relationship to social dis-courses. It is also, at the same time, a guide to how the therapist can approach obtaining the story of the abuse from family members. When families enter therapy, they do so with a dominant account of their history of relationships in which the abuse may be presented as a central or as an insignificant part. By unpacking their story using a genealogical lens, we embark on a rewriting of their history, a rewriting that has a more direct relationship to family members' experiences of power and powerlessness both within the past and in the present.

OBTAINING THE STORY OF THE ABUSE

Discussions concerning "abuse" may elicit defensiveness from parents who interpret interest in the incidents of abuse as either evidence of the therapist's alliance with the Department or as an attempt to judge and shame them. For this reason, it is important that the parents are given the space to tell their "story"—the series of events in which the alleged act of abuse is one link in the chain. We use the word "story" here, recognizing that in this context, what the parents tell us may be "only one side of the story," the side that justifies and defends their behavior or position, and that leaves out elements that may be either known or unknown to them.

Creating the space for parents to tell their story is important in several ways. First, when parents are allowed to give reasons for their abusive behavior or, alternatively, claim that they had no control, they are allowed to save face to some degree. When responded to with curiosity and understanding, their defensiveness is lessened, and they are enabled to examine their own behavior and situation more openly. Second, when parents define the problem in their own terms, we are given access to any inherent motivation to change their relationships. Last, and most important, it is through sensitive tracking and unraveling of the *genealogy* of relationships that underpin the story of abuse, that we can begin to deconstruct the dominant accounts in order to make space for the *hidden accounts* that ultimately provide a full and complex accounting for the abuse.

Even when an incident of abuse is the reason that a family was referred to therapy, abuse is not always identified by the parents as either "abusive" or, indeed, as the primary problem. Their concerns may fall into one of three categories: (1) They may only be concerned about the involvement of the Department or professionals, or about an order to attend therapy; (2) their concerns may center around some other behavior or relationship; the abusive incident may be perceived as the straw that broke the camel's back, perhaps precipitating the family into therapy but, nevertheless, only as a symptom of long-standing relationship problems or the parents' difficulties in managing a child's behavior; (3) the abuse may be acknowledged and presented as *the problem*. Other problems may or may not also be acknowledged.

The degree to which parents perceive their behavior as abusive, and the extent to which they are initially able to take responsibility for their behavior, will become apparent by what the parents define as the problem when they first enter therapy. Their description of the "problem" will reflect the degree to which they experience or perceive the abuse as within the volition of the abuser, and the degree to which they think the abuse is "wrong," that is, as contradictory to the values inherent in the discourse in which they operate. Some parents, for example, make no attempt to deny their actions but, rather, justify their behaviors as is the case, for example, of parents who believe in severe physical discipline:

> The Department referred Sally Travis, a single-parent mother of four children, to therapy when they discovered that she had severely beaten her 10-year-old daughter. The Department defined the problem as one of physical abuse. Sally defended and justified her action on the basis that Allison had been getting into serious trouble and had been stealing desperately needed money from her purse. She believed that Allison's behavior had been influenced by a "naughty" girl at school who had a history of getting into trouble.

The abuse may be justified as common cultural practice. The parents' view of "normal" may or may not differ from the well-functioning members of the same cultural/ethnic group. It is important, therefore, that therapists learn about the cultural practices of their client groups before beginning work with them (Lau, 1986).

Other parents express remorse and describe their behavior as out of kilter with what they believe they want or should be doing within their relationships. Acts of physical and sexual abuse are described as arising from a compulsion or uncontrollable reaction. Although they might respond defensively and rationalize their behavior when confronted, these parents are critical and ashamed of what they have done and feel unable to account for it.

> John Orczy sexually assaulted his daughters over several years. He expressed remorse and shame, and had no explanation for why he had done so. He described the assaults as a compulsion over which he had no control.

It is most likely that there will be multiple contradictions and conflicts within the story initially given by the parents. In those situations where both parents present similar accounts, it is important to remember that the nonabusing parent may have adapted through threat, intimidation, or fear of loss to the abusive parent's perspective. Even for the abuser, however, the picture is rarely so straightforward. A father, for example, who initially justifies his behavior and presents himself as hard and unfeeling, may not show a softer, more vulnerable side that has been repressed in the interests of the dominant discourses within the family and social contexts. On the other hand, a father who claims "no control" over his abusive behavior and appears ashamed and remorseful may not initially reveal another part of himself, currently outside of his conscious awareness, a part for whom the abuse was a purposeful and directed activity, a tactic within a relationship struggle (see Chapter 5). These are the gaps, the hidden accounts, that successful therapy may bring forth.

It is important to actively solicit a definition of the problem from every person present and not simply accepts the mother's or father's definition as speaking for the family as a whole. By assuming that there are conflicts of interest and perspective, the therapist can actively seek out these differences.

In exploring the concerns of other family members, it may be found that they define the problem as a parent's abusive behavior, or that they are more concerned about some other behavior or relationship. In situations where parents justify their own behavior, children may describe themselves as the problem, accepting that they invite the abuse. Alternatively, depending upon their freedom to do so and the degree to which their account remains hidden even from themselves, they may challenge this view.

The following case examples demonstrate the range of concerns that may be identified by other family members:

In the case of the Travis family, Allison, 10, who had been beaten by her mother after several episodes of stealing from her mother's purse, was quiet and withdrawn during the session. When asked about her concerns she answered, "I don't know" to most questions, ultimately saying that the problem was that she was "naughty" and couldn't help getting into trouble. Her sister and brother said the problem was that Allison was always fighting with them and getting into trouble with their mother.

Rita Orczy, the wife of John, who had sexually assaulted their daughters over several years, said she was angry and outraged about the abuse. She had no understanding of why it had happened and wanted it to never happen again. She described how, over 19 years, she had lived in fear of John's moody disposition and that both she and the children had for years done much to placate him and avoid his angry outbursts. She nevertheless said she loved John and did not want the marriage to end. Her daughters, aged 17 and 16, were relieved that the situation had been brought to light, and that the abuse had stopped. They did not want the abuse to begin again and, like their mother, were intimidated by their father's moody nature and frequent angry outbursts.

Fatima Nicolopoulos was distraught to learn about the sexual abuse of her daughter, 16, by her husband. From her perspective, however, it was not out of character with him, and she perceived this problem as one of many in their family relationships. She described him as controlling, intimidating, and verbally abusive. The children described being afraid of their father's verbal intimidation and violent outbursts. They were aligned with their mother and angry with their father both for the abuse and for his extreme control over their activities outside the home.

As is evident in these case examples, family members may experience the abuse as less of a problem than the associated verbal abuse, betrayal, intimidation, and control.

The next task is to locate the range of family members' concerns within a temporal–material context, that is, eliciting their story of "what happened" in terms of behaviors, actions, and events as they unfolded over time.

This may be done by exploring the first known occasion when the abuse occurred. There are often two "onsets" to the problem: the onset of the abuse, and the onset of the relationship struggles that, some way down the track, eventuate in the behavior defined as abusive. Their perceptions of the circumstances and major life events contributing to changes in relationships can then be tracked. The interlocking stories and perceptions of events surrounding episodes of abuse will indicate areas of underlying struggles and thus the relationship context.

As therapists, we often perceive a situation as more optimistic if the parents appear remorseful for their abusive behavior. Taking responsibility for the harmful impact one has on another person, however, is multifaceted. There are at least five aspects to a genuine "taking of responsibility" (see Table 9.1), and most clients entering therapy have gaps in at least a few of these areas.

Taking responsibility in the fullest sense means that first, the parents acknowledge having committed the behavior and both perceive and acknowledge that the behavior was "wrong." Second, the parents understand and acknowledge their own underlying interpersonal reasons for their actions (in terms of their feelings of anger, hurt, sense of unfairness, desire to retaliate, i.e., their "hidden accounts"). Third, rather than denying or minimizing the consequences of their actions, the parents recognize and appreciate the destructive effects of their behaviors. Last,

TABLE 9.1. Aspects of Responsibility

Responsibility	Denial of responsibility
1. Accept and acknowledge that the behavior is wrong.	Deny having committed the behavior or justify the behavior.
2. Understand and acknowledge own interpersonal reasons for behavior (hidden account).	Claim to have no control or give a false or superficial account or rationalization.
3. Recognize and appreciate the interpersonal impact of the behavior and its destructive effects on others.	Blame others. Fail to see how others are responding to oneself.
4. Reinterpret the meaning of others' actions (revelation of others' hidden accounts).	Deny the harmful effects of the abuse. Fail to understand the effects of the abuse on others.
5. Feel and express remorse for harm done.	Refuse to take a one-down position in relation to family members or authorities.

the parents feel and express remorse for the effects of their behaviors and are able to apologize. Resolution also requires that the parents understand why others acted as they did (i.e., that the parents have access to others' "hidden accounts").

To effect a change intra- and interpersonally that can be sustained outside of therapy and without constant vigilance, therapy must minimally ensure that each of these areas is addressed. As is evident in the following case examples, by beginning with the parents' story of the abuse, it is possible to ascertain the extent to which they are able to take responsibility, the gaps that exist in their ability to do so, and the processes that must be undertaken to fill the remaining gaps.

CASE EXAMPLE: THE ORCZY FAMILY

The Orczy family sought therapy after a family crisis in which John confessed to his wife that he had sexually assaulted their daughters, Leanne, 17, and Sandy, 16, over a period of years. He had ceased assaulting Leanne 2 years ago and Sandy only a few months ago. Over the last several months, Sandy had become increasingly difficult at home and in trouble at school. John, believing the abuse was the cause of her behavior, told his wife that he had sexually abused her. Two younger brothers had not been abused and, up until the father's disclosure, were unaware that their sisters had been abused.

We held three initial meetings. The first was with the parents, John and Rita. The second was with the sisters alone, and the third was with all the siblings. In the initial meetings, we found out the nature of the abuse, determined the extent to which Sandy and Leanne were currently at risk, and the circumstances under which we would undertake therapy with the family.

The daughters described sexual abuse consisting of their father touching them on the genitals while he masturbated against them, stopping short of penetration. It had taken place during the night and occurred intermittently over several years. Both daughters maintained that they were safe now that the secret was out in the open. They described their mother as protective and supportive, and said they would have no hesitation in going to her if they ever felt afraid again. The mother, the daughters, and the sons defined the problem as both sexual abuse and the intimidation family members experienced when subjected to their father's "moods." Although the daughters were over the age at which notification to the CP Department was necessary, we explored with them the option of bringing charges against their father. They were against doing so and were committed to undertaking therapy for themselves and their family.

We proceeded with the therapy by meeting with the daughters and the parents separately for several sessions before bringing them together in family sessions. The following discussion is drawn from the meetings with the parents in which the therapist elicited from the couple their story about the abuse.

In the initial meeting with the couple, John defined the problem as the sexual abuse and his fear of losing relationships with his wife and children now that the abuse had been disclosed. Although ashamed and remorseful, John could only explain his sexual assault of his daughters as a "compulsion" over which he had little control. Consistent with other family members' complaints about him, he described himself as "moody" and believed that his moods had something to do with his background. His wife, Rita, also subscribed to this view. This definition of the problem was thus the dominant account as it was first presented.

At this stage, it was clear that John could admit his behavior and acknowledge that it was wrong. He was also expressing remorse. He had little understanding of his own interpersonal reasons for the abuse, however, and, instead, presented as having no volition. His "compulsion" was out of his control, and he could give no account of why he acted as he did. It was important, therefore, to locate his behavior within a temporal–material context from which his hidden account could be elicited.

The therapist proceeded to explore John's account of his "moods." When asked for a recent example of his moodiness, John described how he became moody after a frustrating day at work, dealing with other men. He came home in a "bad mood" and remained angry at home or work for some days until Rita started to "kid him around" by talking to him and placating him. The therapist then linked the problem of his moods with his compulsion to sexually abuse.

THERAPIST: And so, what would your feelings have been then if this had happened a few months ago, before you stopped abusing Sandy?

JOHN: Highly sexed. By the end of the week, I did feel highly sexed. Beginning of the week, I didn't feel that way. I didn't know if at the beginning of the week I'd blocked it out or what, but I didn't feel it then.

RITA: I've had a lower back problem, which the doctor says is due to stress. And it's very painful. I couldn't sit down properly, and I couldn't sleep properly.

JOHN: So I knew that Rita wasn't really feeling well enough to have a [sexual] relationship, but I still felt sort of rejected. So, then, I get this sexual feeling toward the end of the week.

THERAPIST: So you felt a bit rejected by Rita. And did that feeling of rejection happen before or after getting that feeling of feeling highly sexed?

JOHN: Well, it happened before. Even starting at the beginning of the week, I felt a little bit rejected.

THERAPIST: And how did you feel that Rita was rejecting you?

JOHN: Well, I sort of felt rejected by her and I didn't. I sort of had that feeling like when Rita used to be really so tired with the children that she couldn't be bothered with me. I would sort of touch her when she was asleep, and she would sort of pull away, which I think is a natural thing if you're asleep. But I used to get a bit angry about that.

THERAPIST: And what do you do when you're feeling highly sexed and Rita for some reason does not?

JOHN: Well, I just frequently masturbate, like twice in the morning.

THERAPIST: And when you do masturbate, does that decrease the feeling for a while or increase it?

JOHN: It does decrease it for a while, but then I get a revolting feeling. Like I feel dirty. To me, it's not a normal act and I sort of feel disgusted with myself, but then by the time I get to work, I sort of feel it all again, and I have to masturbate again.

THERAPIST: So when you're feeling highly sexed, how many times a day would you have to masturbate?

JOHN: It could be three to five times a day. Sometimes only once and then I think to myself, "This is silly." And I try to control myself, but it's the same sort of feeling like I got with the girls. I didn't want to do it, but I had to do it. And I don't know why.

THERAPIST: So if this had been a couple of years ago, instead of now, and you were feeling that highly sexed feeling, what would have you done? Would you have masturbated or would you have gone into the girls' room, or==

JOHN: ==Probably a mixture of both. I often used to start to masturbate in the bed, but if Rita would start to wake up and I'd get interrupted, I would think, "Bugger this," and I would get up and go and see one of my daughters. That's how it started off then. And then there was times that I would masturbate so many times that I didn't want to have sex with her. I would be impotent.

RITA: Since we've been married, he's had a lot of problems in that department.

JOHN: What would disturb me a lot is that even after masturbating, I would still have that feeling, and I might want to go and see my daughter. Sometimes I would still have that feeling after I had sex with Rita. And that would disturb me, because I would think, "I've just had relations with my wife!" Sometimes I would go for a long time, sometimes even several months, and then, all of a sudden, it would all happen again.

RITA: Our whole married life it's been like we might have sex regularly for quite a while, and then, all of a sudden, he just chops it off, and he won't come near me for months. Even if I try to, you know, initiate, he would say, "No, I'm going to be impotent," and I used to get the feeling that he was trying to punish me. One time we had been having sex regularly and enjoying it. And then I remember one time, when one night I didn't want to because I wasn't feeling well, and I said to him, "Love, do you mind if we don't, and we can tomorrow night?" and he said, "No, now we won't have sex for months. And it doesn't matter what you do to me to try to make me have sex, you won't get sex." And I would say, "Fair enough," but I was just as stubborn as he was.

THERAPIST: When you did have periods where you had sex regularly and enjoyed it, how often would you have it?

RITA: Every night.

JOHN: Every night, and then, suddenly, I would just switch off.

RITA: I would like it before I went to sleep, and John would like it at one or two in the morning, when I was absolutely dead!

JOHN: I go to bed early and then sometimes in the middle of the night I wake up. I would be wide awake, just as I am now, and I would feel aroused.

RITA: I would be too tired. I'd be really asleep then. And that's when he'd feel really rejected.

THERAPIST: What sorts of meanings does it have for you to have sex with Rita?

JOHN: Well sometimes it means love, and I get a very sort of special feeling with her. Other times, it's a mixture of hate and lust, and it becomes just performing the sex act for my own satisfaction. . . . I don't know why, but sometimes I have a sort of a fear that someone will walk in the room and sort of attack me. I always have that feeling that I might be in the process of, you know, sort of being vulnerable to someone coming in. I don't know why. I've just had that feeling. Just sort of the door would burst open, and someone would come in and attack me. And I would start to have an aggressive feeling about that.

THERAPIST: In your fantasy, who would it be that would attack you?

JOHN: I don't know. It would just be some stranger, some man who would just come in and perpetrate that. It would be an unknown person.

In this section of the interview, it appeared to us that in some way John linked sex and aggression, and sex and rejection. His "frustration" with other men initiated his anger, which became focused as sexual desire. When his sexual overtures were rejected, his anger and, consequently, his sexual desire increased. His fantasy of being attacked also raised the question of whether he himself had been sexually abused. We inquired about the possible meanings of John's sexual behavior by asking him about his relationship with other men and women, and about his life as a child.

John told the story of his life, beginning with how he was born in Europe during World War II. When the city in which his family was living was bombed, his parents sent his older brother and sister away to live in the countryside. Born toward the end of the War, John was allowed to stay with his parents. When John was 3, his great aunt moved into the family home, where she spent the last 6 months of her life. He shared a room with her and recalled experiencing her as the "one loving person" in his life. After her death, his mother went out to work and frequently left John alone all day, locked in the kitchen.

When his siblings returned, his older brother was jealous and angry. Perceiving John as receiving preferential treatment from their father, the brother intimidated and at times physically assaulted John. When John was 8 years old, his brother began sexually harassing and then assaulting him. John remembered clearly how, on one occasion, his brother tried to force him to have oral sex. John refused, and the brother slapped him. Although the commotion attracted the attention of his father, John protected his brother and refused to tell his parents, fearing that his often-violent father would "really kill" the brother. In putting together these significant pieces of the puzzle of John's past, we were able to construct with John how, through an emotionally significant relationship of power, John came to associate sex with aggression, power, and powerlessness.

As a small and slightly built man, John said he'd always felt threatened by other men, both physically and sexually, and he frequently felt rejected by women. In his late teens, he immigrated to Australia for a better life but felt lost and lonely away from his family, and rejected and misunderstood by his workmates at the factory where he found work. He had difficulty meeting women in his late teens and early 20s. Rita was his first significant relationship. Rita had been married previously, when she was 18, a marriage precipitated by an unplanned pregnancy, which she subsequently miscarried. She left this relationship after a year of being physically and sexually abused. John and Rita, married and soon thereafter, their baby, Leanne, was born. Two years later, they had a son, Jason, followed 2 years later by another son, Daryl.

Shortly after Jason's birth, Sandy, Rita's 3-year-old niece, was orphaned when her teenage mother was killed in a motor-vehicle accident. She came to live with John and Rita, and was formally adopted by them. Although John was happy to have a family of his own and had agreed without hesitation to the adoption, he was unprepared for Rita's total involvement with the children and found himself once again facing feelings of exclusion and rejection, feelings that were compounded when Sandy came to live with them. Recalling how Sandy had seemed to reject John's attempts to be friendly, Rita explained that Sandy had been "shifted from pillar to post" between grandparents and relatives after her mother's death. She was insecure and clung to Rita, and Rita, in turn, felt a great compassion for, and connection with, her orphaned niece.

John's unacknowledged feelings of being excluded could be seen to constitute one aspect of a hidden account, his unacknowledged, interpersonal reasons for why he acted as he did.

THERAPIST: You seem to make some connection concerning Sandy coming into the family and feeling left out?

JOHN: Yes, I thought that Rita was more intense with Sandy than with me. But I think it was just a figment of my imagination.

THERAPIST: But you were a bit jealous of her relationship with Sandy.

JOHN: Yeah, because that seemed to be the run of my life, actually, always getting left out. And here I'd sort of met a girl at last where we just seemed to sort of click. And I loved her because she was the only woman, really the only person, who ever really sort of treated me right. So I sort of felt threatened when Sandy came and demanded all the attention. She didn't seem to want to be friendly with me; she just wanted to push me away. At the time, I was very angry with her, and I used to be a bit on the cruel side to her sometimes. Tease her a lot, that's how it started.

THERAPIST: What sense did you make of it?

JOHN: I enjoyed being a bit cruel, I really did. I'm ashamed to say it, but I really did. I enjoyed it. I got a certain satisfaction, I guess, because she was rejecting me. At the time, I seemed to get a bit of excitement, a bit of sexual excitement out of it, just to see the fear in her.

THERAPIST: And then, when did it start to become more sexual?

JOHN: It wouldn't have been long after that. Around the time that Daryl was born. Sandy was about 5.

THERAPIST: Let me just try to understand. It's obviously complicated, because you were feeling angry with her as well as wanting her to love you. So I'm just trying to sort through those things. So when it started to become more sexual, what did you do?

As a European migrant who spoke with an accent, John felt less accepted and less acceptable in what, at that time, was still a predominantly "white" (WASP) Australia. Within a culture in which masculinity is constructed in terms of physical strength and sexual prowess, John also fared badly. His masculinity was constantly challenged and found to be inadequate by both men and women. As a working-class man, he was limited to a narrow range of emotional expression. Anger and sexual desire were acceptable masculine feelings, but hurt and vulnerability were not. John expected that his wife would, and should, satisfy his sexual "needs." His "needs," however, were overwhelming, because they were complicated and compounded by his need to belong, his need to be confirmed as masculine, as adequate in relation to the men at work. To receive the almost unhoped for validation and love from a woman made him precariously dependent on her. To then be rejected by her felt intolerable and confirmed the world's perception of him as unmanly and inadequate.

Through the therapist's questions, John revealed aspects of his experience (i.e., his hidden account of the relationship struggles at that time). He, however, demonstrated little understanding or appreciation of the effects of his behavior on a young child. In fact, he seemed to perceive the child as just as vulnerable and perhaps more powerful than himself.

John recalled how he periodically took Sandy for a car ride and had her engage in touching him genitally. This would sometimes occur every day for a week, and then "the feeling would go away," and he would not do it again for some months. Rita added that Sandy had become fond of John and often followed him around.

THERAPIST: John, once you made your relationship with Sandy sexual, what effect did it have on those feelings of being rejected?

JOHN: I felt closer toward Sandy, and I started to feel a bit more angry toward Rita, especially if she was feeling too tired to have sex with me.

THERAPIST: What sense did you make of her being too tired to have sex with you?

JOHN: She was expecting the children, but I didn't really understand. I thought that she should be still interested in me.

THERAPIST: And at that time, did it seem fair or unfair to you that she didn't want to have sex as often as you did?

JOHN: Well to me, then, it did seem unfair. I finally found this woman that I thought really loved me. I married her to be with her. And then it seemed like she had no time for me. I would work all day and come home to feel like a nobody.

THERAPIST: Rita, do you think that by making things sexual with Sandy, John was finding a way of punishing Sandy for getting between you and him, or more finding a way to punish you for making him feel like a nobody when he really loved you?

RITA: Well, he did really hurt Sandy. But he could not have found a better way to hurt me as well. He could not have hurt me more than by doing what he did to the girls.

THERAPIST: What do you think, John? Was it more a way of punishing Sandy or more a way of punishing Rita?

JOHN: That's a hard question to answer. A bit of both, I guess. I didn't know how to make it any better with Rita. I felt really upset, angry a lot of the time. I know it wasn't right, what I did, but I did feel like it was unfair that I got left out.

Out of his anger at feeling rejected, John acts in a revengeful and destructive way—he attempts to have power *over* in order to reduce his own feelings of powerlessness. As a working-class man, John believed that in marrying Rita, he had entered a bargain. That bargain was that he would sacrifice his life through working at hard, demeaning labor in order to support his wife and their children in exchange for the love of a woman who would nurture and validate him. But shortly after marrying, John discovered that his relationship with Rita was not to be an exclusive one. The children came between him and his greatest source of validation and nurturance—his sexual relationship with Rita was often unavailable.

John had little recognition and appreciation, however, of the meaning of Rita's actions or the unfairness to Rita of her end of the "bargain." She found herself in the situation of unending domestic labor, chronic tiredness, and the expectation that she alone care for their children and her father, and that she do all of this without recognition because she was a woman. Rita, herself, while at some level experiencing the unfairness of her position, also felt that she had little to complain about. Marriage and motherhood were her life.

THERAPIST: And what about for you, Rita? What do you remember it being like for you in those first few years?

RITA: Well, I didn't know what was happening. I knew how mean John could get when he was teasing Sandy. I thought it was a bit strange. I was starting to realize that there was something wrong in his background.

THERAPIST: And what was it like for you in getting married?

RITA: We had only been married about 3 weeks when my mother died and father started living with us. And he stayed with us for 6 years, and in that time, we had three babies and adopted Sandy. So we never really had much time to ourselves then. We've never really had time on our own, ever. And I guess for somebody like John, that would be a bit hard to take.

THERAPIST: Your father came to live with you and you had *four* children in 6 years.

RITA: Yeah, that's right. It was a lot to manage at that time.

THERAPIST: How was it decided that your father would live with you?

RITA: Well, he didn't cope after my mother died, and there really was no place else for him to go. John said he could stay with us for a while.

THERAPIST: And how did the two of you work out the labor around the house? There would be a lot to do to care for four children and three adults. Who did all the work?

RITA: Well, John mowed the lawn and took care of the car, but it was really up to me to do everything else. John worked, and he was tired when he got home. My father helped some, but he didn't have much patience with the children.

THERAPIST: And how tired were you?

RITA: I would fall into bed at night too tired to move, and then I would have to get up during the night to the baby. I tried to be interested in sex for John, but sometimes I just couldn't.

THERAPIST: And were you tired because, as John said, you were pregnant, or because of the heavy work load you carried every day?

RITA: Well, it was both. Not just that I was pregnant. I never had a chance to stop or rest. John could never understand that. He didn't know how much work it was to keep the whole house going. He couldn't understand why I got so tired looking after the kids and my father.

THERAPIST: You must have been exhausted. Did it feel fair or unfair to you that the entire workload fell on your shoulders?

RITA: I thought it was my job. I didn't think I had any right to complain. At times I would think, "Why do I have to do all this? What have I got myself into?"

By obtaining the story of abuse, this interview was a beginning in identifying the gaps in John's initial ability to take responsibility for the abuse. It was also a beginning in outlining the content of these gaps: John's sensitivity to rejection, his retaliation for perceiving himself as left out and rejected, his lack of understanding of the position of Sandy or the unfairness of Rita's position. The interview was brought to an end by the therapist summarizing the interview. She empathized with John's pain, validated his feelings of rejection and exclusion, and underlined that his "compulsion" which, perhaps until now, was "unconscious," was in fact a choice of retaliation to "right" what he perceived as the unfairness of his position. The therapist then empathized with Rita for the sacrifices she had made and the unfairness of the expectations laid on her as a wife and mother, and of the unfairness of John's retaliation, the ultimate betrayal of her trust in John, and the pain he had brought to her children.

CASE EXAMPLE: THE TRAVIS FAMILY

In the case that follows, the mother did not acknowledge or accept that her behavior constituted abuse or "was wrong," nor did she initially appear to feel or express remorse for any wrongdoing. These aspects of "taking responsibility" were made possible only after the therapy had made accessible her daughter's hidden account that explained to the mother the daughter's misbehavior in a dramatically new way and thus allowed the mother to recognize and appreciate the impact of her behavior on her daughter. The following transcript of the second session of the Travis family illustrates well the process of unpacking and rewriting the story.

Sally Travis was the sole parent of four children—Danny, 14, Susan, 11, Allison, 10, and Rick, 8. Two years ago, she left her violent husband to live with the children in public housing, supported by a sole-parent benefit. The children had no contact with their father.

Sally and her children were ordered by the Court to attend family therapy after the Department had placed Allison in temporary foster care. In making the referral, the CP Worker explained that Allison had run away from home after being beaten by her mother. When the Department contacted her mother, Sally said she did not want Allison at home, because she had been stealing.

In the second session, we elicited from family members the story of the abuse. The dominant account, given by Sally, described how Allison had turned "naughty," eventually stealing money after becoming involved with a "bad girl" at school named Mary Anne. Sally said she had beaten Allison to "try to get through to her" and convince her to behave. Allison had been stealing $20 notes from her mother's purse on several occasions. This was money the family could not afford to lose. Sally did not claim to have lost control when she abused her daughter. She acknowledged that she beat Allison, but she justified doing so on the grounds that under the circumstances, it was necessary and appropriate discipline. It was the Department, not Sally, who defined her behavior otherwise.

In the session, Allison was quiet and withdrawn, eventually saying only that the problem was that she was naughty. Susan and Danny were clearly aligned against Allison. They described her as "naughty" and said that they did not miss having her at home. Things were better without her, they said, because Allison provoked many fights with them and with their mother.

In tracking the episode in which Sally had beaten Allison and the problem of Allison stealing, the siblings' perception of the time when Allison began taking money was elicited:

SUSAN: Sometimes she was throwing it out the door, and sometimes she was throwing it out my bedroom window. My bedroom has no screen; all of the other windows have. So sometimes she was throwing it out my bedroom window.

THERAPIST: How did you know she was doing it?

SUSAN: I didn't know, but my brother did, because he used to get up to go to the toilet. She used to open my curtain so that Danny would think that I took the money.

THERAPIST: Why do you think that she threw it out your window? Why would she want to make it look like you did it?

SUSAN: I don't know. Oh, yes, I do. She thought that Mum wasn't taking her out and everything. She wouldn't give Allison ice cream if she was giving us ice cream if Allison had been into it the night before.

Susan related how when "we" (Susan and her mother) visited the neighbors next door, Allison, left home alone, would eat massive amounts of ice cream and peanut butter. The mother replied that this was "throwing money away." Food that was supposed to last a week, Allison consumed in one sitting. At this stage, it was evident that Allison was excluded from important family relationships, a situation likely to elicit feelings of hurt and powerlessness.

The therapist began to explore the history of relationship struggles by beginning with how the mother believed Mary Anne, the "naughty" girl at the school, fit into the picture. Sally described how she had heard through the teacher of Mary Anne's reputation for troublemaking, and she had told the children not to play with her. Allison had rebelled and insisted on playing with the girl. Susan then told the story of how Mary Anne had tried to steal her best friend. When Susan won back her best friend, together they rejected Mary Anne, who said that she would then become friends with Allison.

THERAPIST: How did you see the relationship between these two [sisters] before Mary Anne came on the scene?

MOTHER: Good . . . as close as any other sisters. They used to play together at school. I thought that both of them were playing with Mary Anne.

THERAPIST: Do you agree with that? Did you think that you were pretty good buddies with your sister?

Allison: (*nodding yes, vigorously*) Yeah.

THERAPIST: And do you agree with that?

SUSAN: Hmm.

THERAPIST: As time has gone on, have you gotten to be better buddies or worse buddies?

SUSAN: Worse.

In tracking back the genealogy of relationships in this case, the first point of conflict relating to the aforementioned was identified as the issue concerning the children's choice of friends. Both Sally and the teachers held the dominant position that Mary Anne was a "naughty" girl who could influence Sally's children negatively. When Sally issued the injunction that the children not play with Mary Anne, Susan complied, but Allison resisted and became friends with Mary Anne anyway. What was not acknowledged or validated within the mother's account was that Allison was a shy girl with difficulties making friends, and that her situation was exacerbated by having a more outgoing, articulate, and competitive older sister within the same peer group. Allison, feeling both excluded and powerless to compete with Susan, aligned with Mary Anne.

The next point of conflict between Allison and her mother was related to an incident in which Allison had pushed Susan over while Susan was rollerskating, resulting in Susan seriously scraping one of her arms. Susan had been playing with Allison's "old boyfriend." Although Susan maintained that Allison had already "dropped him," Allison indicated that this was not so.

THERAPIST: So what was it like for you? You thought you hadn't dropped him. What was it like for you seeing your sister play with him?

ALLISON: I was jealous.

THERAPIST: Do you think Susan gets jealous of Allison as well?

MOTHER: In some cases, yes, I think Allison reacts, um, Allison reacts a lot, whereas with Susan, she takes it on. Whereas with Susan, she handles it. You don't see it as much. I think she would be, but she doesn't make it as obvious.

THERAPIST: So do you two think you got to be less good buddies since this incident with the rollerskates?

Both say: Mm.

THERAPIST: After that, how did she act toward you? Was she still nice to you, or did she give you the cold shoulder?

ALLISON: She used to . . . ignore me.

THERAPIST: How did Susan respond to her?

MOTHER: Well, I didn't think that she was.

THERAPIST: How did Allison respond to Susan?

MOTHER: Very spiteful.

THERAPIST: Did you have any ideas at that time what it was about?

MOTHER: No, I didn't really know what it was about. Allison, from that time, really, from that time, she was nasty toward all of us. She sort of changed within herself.

THERAPIST: What sense did you make of that.

MOTHER: Well, see, the rollerskating incident and the money missing was about the same time. . . . I felt it was more tied in with the Mary Anne incident.

THERAPIST: Did you think that Susan wanted you to be buddies with her after that?

ALLISON: No (*shaking her head*).

THERAPIST: Did you think that Allison wanted to be buddies with you after that, or not?

SUSAN: She did, but I didn't want to after what had happened. Because I was really screaming . . . and I came in, and blood was coming off my arms.

THERAPIST: How did your mum respond?

ALLISON: She was mad.

Susan then vividly described the injuries to her knees and elbows. In doing so, she earned her mother's intense attention, while Allison put her hand on her chin and looked the other way.

THERAPIST: Who do you think the girls would say has been closest to you? I know that it changes over time with kids.

MOTHER: Ah, well I have no favoritism among any of the children. I try to treat them all the same, because I don't feel any different to Susan than I do toward Allison.

THERAPIST: Of course, but they will often feel it differently, even though the parent does not intend it that way.

MOTHER: Yeah.

THERAPIST: Allison, who do you think your Mum is closest to out of all the kids?

ALLISON: Them—those three.

Conflict between sisters over friends was enacted again in the incident in which Susan "stole" Allison's boyfriend, again excluding Allison and demonstrating her social superiority. Susan defined the relationship between Allison and her "boyfriend" as "over." Allison's hidden account centered around her feelings of jealousy, rejection, and need to belong. But these were experiences she could not acknowledge or discuss. Such discussions were not part of the discourse of this family. Instead, Allison chose to resist by retaliating and pushing Susan over while rollerskating. While this was obviously a physically painful episode for Susan, she used it to her advantage within the sisters' struggle over position in relation to their mother. Unaware of what lay behind Allison's actions, their mother was horrified that Allison would deliberately cause Susan these injuries and attributed her behavior to the influence of the "naughty girl," Mary Anne. She defined Allison as "bad" and aligned with Susan. Allison's hurt and anger, her experience of unfairness and injustice, were subjugated and lost. The dominant account held that Sally was "fair" with all of her children and did not give preferential treatment. Only Allison perceived it differently. When Susan was asked who her mother was closest to, she replied, "The whole mob." When Allison was asked how things were different 6 months ago, before the problem, in terms of her closeness to her mother, she said it was different but couldn't describe how.

THERAPIST: Before Allison left the house, who do you think between you and Allison missed your friendship the most? Like when you two became not such good buddies?

SUSAN: Well, I didn't like it either, but I think that she missed it.

THERAPIST: How could you tell?

SUSAN: I wasn't talking to her very much 'cause of what she did.

THERAPIST: Who would you say missed the friendship the most?

ALLISON: I don't know (*looking away*).

When asked about Mary Anne, Allison said she had made friends with Mary Anne because she had difficulty making friends at school. This was unlike Susan, who had many friends at school. Sally added that "Allison is not as outgoing as Susan."

THERAPIST: What about in the family? Is that true in the family as well? Was Susan more outgoing than Allison?

MOTHER: Probably, yeah.

THERAPIST: So, Susan shines a little bit.

Sally described Susan as "talkative" and, true to form, Susan then gave a detailed description about how she adjusts when she goes to a new school.

THERAPIST: Who do you think Allison takes after?

SALLY: I think she is very much like her father, really.

THERAPIST: And how's her father?

SALLY: He is dark—dark eyes, dark hair. Susan is blonde, like me (*laughs*). I guess in some ways, Allison's like me, but she's also like herself.

Allison felt powerless in relation to her sister, both at home and at school. She began stealing money from her mother. This was not money she used for herself but, rather, she literally threw the money out the window and transparently framed Susan by throwing it out *her* window. In this act, Allison attacked her mother where it hurt the most, at the heart of her mother's inadequate financial situation. Despite the framing of Susan, Sally did not think for a moment that Susan had committed the theft. But this mattered little, for what Allison intended very clearly to communicate was that Susan, as well as her mother, was the objects of her attack.

By stealing, Allison confirmed for Sally her belief that Allison was indeed bad. Her mother asserted this view and attempted to "get through to her" by beating her for the theft. Less acknowledged by Sally and perhaps lying at the heart of her inability to perceive Allison's need to be included and belong was her perception between the similarity between Allison and Allison's father, both in terms of *looks* and *personality*. Perhaps in one way, Sally was wreaking the revenge on Allison that she had been unable to inflict upon her absent ex-husband. In this round of conflict, Allison's need for her mother's love and her experience of exclusion and rejection were subjugated. These needs and desires could not be labeled or expressed. Allison resisted by running away.

In running away, Allison enlarged the scope of the conflict by involving others, in particular, the Department, into the conflict between her mother and herself. This time, the Department had the dominant position. The CP Worker defined Sally rather than Allison as bad, and Allison as the victim of her mother's abuse. The CP Worker attributed Sally's abusive behavior to the abuse Sally herself had suffered as a child.

The CP Worker's position subjugated Sally and her children's experience of their relationship struggles, Sally's despair and frustration at trying to be a good mother and keep her children good, and the meaning to Sally, a single parent of four children living in poverty, of having $20 notes taken from her purse and thrown away. Sally resisted this subjugation in one of the few ways she had left at her disposal—she told the Department to keep Allison. The Department may well have done so had the Magistrate in the Children's Court not ordered them to find therapy for the family.

On one level, the conflicts within the Travis family arose out of the idiosyncratic features of their family life: a single-parent mother overwhelmed by the demands of four children; two daughters close in age, both highly competitive for their mother's attention. Allison felt rejected and powerless to resist this definition of herself in relation to her mother and her sister. She struck at the heart of her mother's greatest sense of powerlessness—to steal money that was desperately needed to buy food for the family.

The fabric of their family life was also interwoven with social discourses concerning motherhood and parent–child relations. The competition between the two sisters reflected the sense of impoverishment and powerlessness within this family, both in terms of material commodities and the availability of adult attention. The social undervaluing of women's work and child care, along with the inability of Sally to secure any employment that could begin to meet their material needs, left the family in a tenuous material existence in which the loss of $20 notes and taking more than one's share of ice cream took on significant meaning.

Sally Travis believed she was responsible (and was perceived by the school as responsible) for keeping her children well behaved and under control. Knowing that she was perceived as a single-parent "welfare" mother, Sally felt pressured to keep Allison under control. Her sense of inadequacy in doing so encouraged her to frame her children's behavior in terms of good and bad, right and wrong. Sally could beat Allison because she felt powerless as a mother to influence her behavior in any other way, and because she felt entitled to do so.

In physically abusing her own daughter, Sally Travis operated from a network of suppositions that reflected commonplace discourses concerning parenting. To be out of control as a parent, from Sally's viewpoint, was a greater failing than having bruised her daughter. Parents must be in control of children and have the right and duty to ensure the child's compliance by physical discipline if necessary. This construction of parent–child relationships in terms of obedience and compliance prevented Sally from seeking information that would allow her to see Allison's behavior in any other light.

CONCLUSION

This chapter demonstrates a method of obtaining the parents' "story" of the series of events in which the alleged abuse is one link in the chain. This story provides the framework from which the therapist can reconstruct the relationship context in which the abuse was perpetrated.

In exploring the multiple layers of unfairness and injustice representing the subjugated, hidden accounts of family members, it is possible to identify how each person expresses his or her resistance. This resistance is directed toward those whose dominant views or behaviors led to the sense of unfairness. In turn, by resisting, the individual behaves in a manner that is perceived by others as unfair or oppressive. This is especially so when the abuser, whose position of power, either as a man or a parent, enables him or her to enforce dominance and redress what is perceived as unfairness in a manner that is ultimately destructive to others and to relationships.

◖◖

Creating a
Relationship Discourse

As we explore and rewrite the story of abuse, a theme repeatedly emerges. Parents who abuse a child often do so after a prolonged period of feeling powerless and unfairly treated themselves. Feeling unable to rectify the situation, they retaliate and attempt to gain power over others through the act of abuse. In doing so, they generate in others another round of hurt, injustice, and, ultimately, resistance. Therapy can point to a different kind of relationship discourse in which family members experience and acknowledge their own hidden thoughts, needs, and desires, develop an ability to listen for and acknowledge the effect of their behaviors on others, and make a commitment to nonviolence and fairness and equity in relationships.

Social discourses demand and create a narrow range of options for relationships and restrain actions and behaviors within them. To act outside of these definitions positions one as deviant: unmasculine, unfeminine, a bad mother, a bad wife. The basic premises underlying these discourses, however, are often in conflict with what individuals need or desire.

On a more personal level, parents, particularly working class parents, often lack the language to conceptualize and talk about their experience of hurt and injustice, or to create the space in which to elicit their partner's or children's experiences. Moreover, there is often little motivation to do either when there has been a history of hurt and unfairness. To make oneself vulnerable, particularly in the presence of those who have treated us unjustly, can be frightening, requiring courage, determination, and a belief in the outcome based on successful experience with the process.

In this approach, the focus on relationships begins in the first session (whether that is focused on the relationship between parents and CP Workers or on intrafamily relationships) and continues to the end of therapy. The conversation that occurs in therapy models how to think and talk about relationships, how to access one's own hidden accounts, and make space for and elicit the accounts of others. A focus on relationships is maintained across sessions by (1) using part of each session to explore perceptions of current relationships and changes in relationships between family members since the last session, and (2) examining problems or issues that arise between sessions by exploring the relationship context in which they occur. This presumes that relationships are fluid and ever changing and that one can never step in the same river twice.

Descriptions of relationships may also be elicited according to particular concepts and values about relationships. Questions, for example, may concern such values as fairness, support, respect, fidelity, loyalty, honesty, integrity, trust, love, commitment, genuineness, authenticity, and obedience. Parents might never have articulated their positions concerning these values to themselves, much less explicated and worked out with their partners what the family's ethical base is.

In asking relationship questions, the therapist remains central, speaking to each person and discouraging interaction between family members. Because family members are often commenting on others rather than themselves, they are intensely interested in what others say, while simultaneously feeling less "on the spot" and less required to justify themselves. This can diffuse potentially volatile situations, giving family members an opportunity to see how they are experienced by others.

When relationships remain the central focus of therapy, the language and concepts that allow relationships to be discussed are introduced. As this occurs over a number of sessions, family members begin to frame their experiences in these terms outside the therapy session and are ultimately able to talk to each other, drawing on this language.

For this different discourse to be incorporated into life outside of therapy, there comes a point at which family members must contact and dialogue with each other directly. In families in which there has been abuse, family members may initially be reluctant to take this step on their own outside of therapy sessions. In such cases, the therapist must become more directive in order to facilitate the needed dialogue between family members. This may happen spontaneously during a session or may be planned and rehearsed to be enacted at a critical stage of therapy that marks change in the nature of relationships.

The third way in which the therapist creates a different form of relationship discourse is by acting as a power broker between family members. This means using the power and influence inherent in the social role of therapists to carefully challenge the dominant discourses by asking questions that carve out a different perspective. At other times, it means selectively using forms of leverage in order to shift the position of family members so that relationship issues can be resolved more fairly.

There are three important areas that therapy must address: a commitment to respect and nonviolence, making apologies a part of the relationship discourse, and facing and resolving relationship issues.

COMMITMENT TO RESPECT AND NONVIOLENCE

One of the first areas for therapy to address is the parents' commitment and, through them, the commitment of other family members to respect and nonviolence in their interactions with each other.

To this end, it is important to fully address the parents' practices concerning physical discipline. Therapy is not successful when it merely shifts parents' behavior from, for example, "beating" or "belting," into open-handed hitting or "smacking," even if the latter is not defined as "abusive" by the CP Department. While the parents are in therapy and motivated, therapy must focus on shifting their values and behaviors away from violent and authoritarian practices. This is done with the knowledge that when therapy and child protection intervention cease and everyday stresses return full blown, it is the parents who are committed to a completely nonviolent approach who are more likely to weather the storm without inflicting further injury to their children.

As described in Chapter 8, therapy should only take place when children are safe from further abuse, and therapy is only likely to be effective when it occurs in a context of sufficient leverage. In a case of physical abuse, a most effective form of leverage early on in therapy is to include the condition that "the parents cease using physical discipline and find alternative ways to discipline" as one of the objectives for therapy (as described in Chapter 7), as prescribed by the CP Department. In those cases in which the Department is not involved at all, the therapist must address the hitting and find intrafamilial forms of leverage to initially restrain the parents. In both cases, however, the therapist must soon move on to eliciting and constructing internal motivation for the parents to stop using physical discipline.

There are three main reasons why it may be in the parents' interests to completely stop using physical discipline and with the therapist's help find other ways of disciplining that they can carry out authoritatively, consistently, and with predictable consequences. For parents who had been investigated by the Department, a most convincing reason is that once "on file," they are likely to remain under the "watchful eye" of the Department. It behooves them to behave in a manner that is beyond reproach. Anything slightly suspicious is likely to be considered (by schools, friends, relatives, and ultimately the CP Department) as evidence of abuse rather than as accidental, and could trigger another course of investigation. When parents stop using physical discipline entirely, they have nothing to defend when a child shows up at school with a bruise.

The other two reasons for parents to stop all physical discipline may not be initially apparent to the parents. Rather, they are elicited and constructed by the therapist by discussing with the parents the consequences of using physical discipline. The first of these has to do with the effect of physical discipline on the parents' relationship with the children. Do the parents want a close and loving relationship with their children, or do they want them to live in fear and intimidation of them? Do they want a child who cooperates with them or a child who puts his or her efforts into opposing and deceiving parents and teachers? The second of these reasons is that, particularly for boys, physical discipline tends to markedly increase their level of aggression at home and outside. Some parents want their children to respect them, and they expect that a necessary component of respect is fear. They are less likely, however, to want a child who is aggressive at home with siblings and in trouble for aggressive behavior at school.

It is often useful to act on the basis that a parent (or at least one of the parents in dual-parent families) will, in fact, agree with one or another of the aforementioned reasons. The therapist then works toward eliciting the parent's agreement to stop using physical discipline. This was the case in the following example of a mother, Jane, her partner, Alan, both in their early 20s, and Jane's preschool children from a previous relationship, Jack and Mandy.

The parents had referred themselves to therapy complaining of the 3-year-old's oppositional behavior and tantrums. Although the mother had had contact with welfare authorities in the past, the family was not currently under investigation. During the first part of the initial interview, the mother and stepfather "smacked" both children several times each while carrying on a conversation with the therapist. The force used against such young children (one who could not even talk, and the other only barely), made the therapist and team members wince. When the therapist commented on the hitting, however, the parents minimized and discounted their behavior and, incredibly to the therapist and team, claimed to believe in "not hitting."

THERAPIST: Jane, I've noticed that you hit Mandy and Jack a number of times today. Would you say this is about how things would go at home?

JANE: Like, well, I just smack her on the hand, I don't, I don't==

ALAN: ==Nothing drastic.

JANE: ==Nothing drastic. I give her a smack on the hand when she doesn't listen to me, and this is why she is a well-behaved child. Very rarely, once in a blue moon, she gets smacked. Once in every few months.

THERAPIST: Oh, I see.

JANE: I don't hit her all the time. She goes to her room if she mucks up. I'll say, "Go to your room," and she'll go to her room (*laughs*). Jack is the type of little kid that doesn't. Why I smacked her was because she's been like Jack a lot, and I don't want him egging her on. She threw something at me, and I don't like that.

THERAPIST: So what you're saying is that you wouldn't normally discipline them like this.

JANE: I rarely, I rarely hit my kids even though Alan does. And I don't hit my kids very often, and when I do it's got to be something that, well, she threw something at me and I want my kids to respect me.

THERAPIST: What about with Jack? What would you do to manage him?

JANE: I put him in his room. I don't hit him. Alan does more smacking than what I do.

ALAN: I don't hit Jack.

JANE: I'm not going to hit him.

ALAN: All I do is point to his room and it's off he goes crying, because I hate hittin' 'im. I hate hittin' kids.

The mother's denial of what just happened in the room was curious. She appeared to know that the therapist would think hitting is wrong, and we suspected she had heard this message before, possibly from the CP Department. Perhaps partly as a way of getting herself off the hook, and partly out of genuine concern for the treatment the child experiences, the mother pointed the finger at the stepfather.

The stepfather, in turn, denied his earlier actions. Rather than confronting him, however, the therapist more neutrally inquired as to why he hated hitting. This had the effect of the stepfather revealing, first, where the parents had received this message before and, second, the extent to which this stepfather had, in fact, abused the 3-year-old.

THERAPIST: Why is that?

ALAN: Well, they say, you know, it shows the kids violence. Like they will end up hitting when they go to school.

THERAPIST: Who would say that?

ALAN: The Welfare and, um, also older people, other parents.

THERAPIST: Would you agree, do you think?

ALAN: I'd agree on it in certain ways, but you have to draw the line with not smacking them. Like I'll admit, yeah, if you start off hitting them, hit them for really bad things and sort of medium-size things and small things they've done, but if you hit 'im all the time, it just ends up monotonous, and they think, "Oh, well, I'll get hit sort of thing," and you don't really worry about it much. I used to hit Jack a fair bit. Like I'd give him a good belting, and he'd come back and do the same thing, and I'd give him another one. It was just like a seesaw.

Although it was evident that the parents had not, in fact, stopped hitting the children, rather than confronting them, the therapist went along with and magnified that part of them that desired not to hit. At the end of the session, the therapist commented on many of the parents' strengths and their honesty and openness in the session, and then positioned himself as aligned with the parents' desire to not use physical discipline. While giving the parents the credit for the reasons for not hitting, the therapist then stated very clearly that he expected all hitting to stop immediately.

THERAPIST: We absolutely agree with you about the hitting. You were saying, Alan, that hitting creates aggressiveness in children, and we absolutely agree with that==

JANE: ==It can.

THERAPIST: ==And we heard what you were saying, Jane, about not wanting Alan to be in the position where he is going to do anything physical like hitting or grabbing Jack, or==

JANE: ==Teasing, or==

THERAPIST: ==Or saying teasing things to him. When people come in to see us, we usually have to tell them to stop doing some of those things==

JANE: ==I'm already stopping.

THERAPIST: We agree with you that hitting can create aggressiveness in kids. And it can make them want to do the opposite of what you want. So their behavior just gets worse and worse. We think you have to make a decision right now that any hitting or anything physical, or any threatening has to stop, and stop now. You've got to make sure that it stops now, and we'll help you find other ways of dealing with the children's behavior.

JANE: I'm just wondering, I'm just wondering if Jack is going to hate Alan toward the end. I don't know.

THERAPIST: We're going to work with you on that.

JANE: I want Jack to love Alan as a father.

ALAN: It's up to her, really.

JANE: It's up to you, too, you know.

Despite the fact that the mother, herself, was also hitting Jack, her greater concern for the effects on Jack provided a beginning point for leverage in getting the parents to stop using physical discipline. It was clear from the mother's expressed concern for the relationship between the stepfather and son that this triangle would have to be addressed and worked out, as it must be in many new stepfamilies. The therapist, however, did not treat the stepfather's violence as a symptom that would fade as the parental conflict decreased and relationships improved. Instead, the therapist ensured that a commitment to nonviolence was put on the agenda in the first session and addressed in every subsequent session.

It was not difficult to move the aforementioned parents into committing themselves to a nonviolent approach because, on the one hand, they were already voicing some, if minimal, movement in that direction. In the following case example, however, the father firmly believed that hitting was an appropriate form of discipline and that it was normal for children to fear their father.

Helen arranged therapy for herself and her husband, Mark, both in their mid-30s, after their reoccurring arguments reached the stage where Helen was considering separating. One of the concerns that Helen expressed in therapy was that Mark hit the children as a form of discipline and that their son, Robbie, 6, had told her repeatedly that he was afraid of his father. In the following segment of the first interview, the therapist attempted to move the father from his position of defending and justifying physical discipline. The therapist had to search through several different possibilities for leverage. Initially, the father resisted fiercely and was not at all responsive to the therapist's attempts to create an opening for change. The parents were argumentative and intense, and frequently spoke over or interrupted each other.

THERAPIST: What sort of a relationship do you want to have with Robbie?

MARK: Um, ah, the one I'm already having, or the one that I *thought* I was having.

THERAPIST: Uh huh. But you found out that he's afraid of you. Do you want him to be afraid of you?

MARK: No, I don't. That's what I said to him on Saturday morning. I said, "There's no point in being frightened of me because I *love* you and, yes, I *do smack* you, but it's what Daddy tries to explain to you, it's what's called 'discipline.' If I think what you're doing is wrong, I'll smack you on the bottom. I'm *not* going to smack you all the time. I'm *not* going to beat you to a pulp or whatever, and there's nothing to be frightened of then." I don't know what Helen is going on about.

The therapist began by searching to create leverage through the father's desire for a good relationship with his son. This was unsuccessful, however, as the father asserted that there was nothing wrong with his relationship with his son. He saw nothing wrong with using smacking as discipline and denied that there was any problem. The therapist then attempted to reestablish the problem in another way by looking at how much his wife trusted him with the children.

THERAPIST: How much do you think that Helen trusts you with the kids? . . . I mean if she was to==

MARK: ==I don't think she trusts me at all. I don't know why. She sees me as a very angry person.

THERAPIST: What do you think *she* would have to see in order to feel like she could trust you?

MARK: Smiling face all the time. A less angry person. I might still be an argumentative person but not, not physically argumentative or anything stupid like that.

THERAPIST: How far away is she from seeing that now, do you think?

MARK: Ah, about a thousand miles. From about here to the equator.

THERAPIST: And how close do *you* feel to it?

MARK: Very, very close.

THERAPIST: How much do you trust Helen with the children?

MARK: Perfectly. I think, ah, the only thing that I would think now, is that she puts the kids through trauma by threatening to break up the family.

THERAPIST: How much do *you* trust Mark with the kids?

HELEN: Not much. I worry about the kids. I know Mark loves them, and he is their father. Um, you know, but I draw the line at some of Mark's methods of discipline. It may be because of what I've read that I believe there are more *effective* ways of disciplining than smacking or threatening to smack. But I don't think it's so much the *smack* that Robbie in particular and Jason to a degree are frightened of, it's the degree to which Mark is out of control of himself that, that frightens them==

MARK: ==That's not true==

HELEN: ==And that does happen==

MARK: ==I've never been out of control. That's just an exaggeration==

HELEN: ==A person who's in complete control of himself doesn't actually put his foot through the kitchen wall==

THERAPIST: ==He does physical things to show his anger.

HELEN: Yeah, if it frightens a *grown-up* who actually, you know, could stand a fairly good chance of defending herself if she really chose to, what does it do to the kids?

THERAPIST: How much do you think Mark's aware of other people feeling intimidated by him? Do you think it's the sort of thing he's aware of?

HELEN: No, he thinks he's Mister Nice Guy, yes. He thinks he's Mister Nice Guy and it's *us* that have a problem. *We* have the problem because we're==

MARK: ==No, I don't.

HELEN: You *imply* it. *We* have the problem because we can't *trust* him, and we don't feel *safe* around him, so it's *our* problem. And but it's *not*; I mean it—it's not *our* problem he's not a person that you could feel safe *around*, because he might let off his temper and he is unpredictable. That is why *I* feel unsafe around him, and why I threaten to leave him.

The problem became one of the mother and children living in fear and intimidation of the father. They did not feel safe. Although the father accused the mother of exaggerating, these concerns could not now be so easily dismissed. The therapist returned to challenging the father to change his behavior by using hypothetical questions, first to the mother, and then to the father.

THERAPIST: Mark obviously loves the children a great deal. Do you think that Mark's love for the kids is such that he could actually, for example, make a resolution to himself that he wouldn't use physical means to discipline?

HELEN: I—I—I don't know that Mark realizes to the extent—I mean, I don't know how or where, I mean, I—I—I'm not really *sure* that he could make that adjustment.

THERAPIST: But say, hypothetically, that he could, OK, then what would that do to your trust in him as a parent?

HELEN: That would help a lot. I could *tell* if he was hitting them when I wasn't there. But if he could actually stop, well, I would know, *for sure*, that when they're in his care, they're safe.

THERAPIST: What about you, Mark. How aware do you think that *you* are at times of whether or not someone feels intimidated by you?

MARK: Ah, oh, *fully* aware. If someone is cringing, you know that they're intimidated. I mean, you've got to be in control of yourself. Oh, I don't know, maybe we weren't made to live together.

Here, the father tried to evade the issue by referring to the possibility of separating. The therapist ignored this and pursued the hypothetical questioning concerning trust.

THERAPIST: Say you *were* to decide that it was very important to you that Helen could feel that she trusted you 100% as a parent and that the children could feel 100% safe with you. If you decided to do that, how easy or hard do you think it would be for you to make a resolution to not smack them or hit other things in their presence?

MARK: That shouldn't be a hypothetical or shouldn't be a debatable point at all because if Helen *can't trust* me to be a good person, to be a good father, then what's the point at all?

THERAPIST: If you were to decide that you wanted to be seen by her as 100% trustworthy and that you wanted Robbie to feel 100% safe with you, how hard or easy would it be for you?

MARK: But why should it be seen by *her*? Why should I make myself that way to her? What, what is she? Lord Almighty God in church?

Again, the father defocused onto the hopelessness of his relationship with his wife. His resistance to his wife defining how he should be prevented him from considering a different approach with his son. The therapist decided to focus solely on his relationship with his son and to use his symmetrical edge to challenge him about whether he was capable of behaving differently with his son.

THERAPIST: Say, then, in terms of your relationship with Robbie, if you were to decide that==

MARK: ==That's why I don't understand the question. I believe that I *do* have a fantastic and very good relationship with my son.

THERAPIST: It sounds like you are very involved and very caring for him, but if, I mean, if for *Robbie's* level of feeling safe with you alone, if that meant that you had to find other ways other than hitting, smacking, or, you know, physical discipline, do you think you would be able to do that, or do you think your anger would be such that it would come out==

MARK: ==Anger's got nothing to do with, because it's past.

THERAPIST: I see.

MARK: Ah, ah, um. I still have very hard . . . I cannot comprehend the question at all. Um, I can understand the *angry* part of it, but I forgot the, but I *can't* understand what==

THERAPIST: ==Could you *decide* to stop hitting him?

MARK: Yes.

THERAPIST: 100%?

MARK: 100%. That would take an effort. I have to say it would take an effort, for the sole reason it's inbred. Just as anger is inbred, especially coming from my background, yeah.

Here, the father softens and gives the therapist an opening—"coming from my background." The therapist, however, misses the chance to explore the meaning of these words and goes one more round with the father before returning to this opening.

THERAPIST: Would you know other ways, or would you have to find other ways?

MARK: I *know*

THERAPIST: I'm not saying it's wrong. But I'm saying that *if* you were to decide that you don't want Robbie to be scared of you==

MARK: ==But *why* is he scared of me? *She* makes him scared of me. Of course, you've got to change your attitudes if a person's actually coming to you saying they're dead scared of you, but he's *not*. My perspective, maybe I've got this totally and utterly wrong, but I think that he's going through what a normal child goes through.

THERAPIST: (*speaking softly*) In my experience, *that is* what normal children whose fathers smack them *do* feel like, but children whose fathers decide *not* to smack them don't feel that way. So, yes, I think it *is* normal.

MARK: *Does that make the child better? For life?* Does that make the child's upbringing better?

THERAPIST: What do you mean by *better?*

MARK: Does that make him a better child ?

THERAPIST: Well, that depends what you define by *better.* If you find other ways to discipline without hitting, usually their behavior is just as good. It probably makes them less aggressive children. Children who don't get smacked don't usually have as much problem with aggression.

MARK: I have to agree with that, because I've got it inbred from the past, and *my* inbreeding from the past wasn't just a smack on the bottom, we got a belt across our legs or a hand across the face for talking out of turn. But that shouldn't carry on. I said to myself from day one of marriage that I would never ever do that to my kids.

THERAPIST: It doesn't sound like you have done it to that extent. You ask me, does it make a better child, and I'm saying that children who get hit tend to become aggressive, and tend to become kids who hit. So it depends on what you want.

MARK: Yeah, I have to agree. I have to agree that I want him to be a better person. I want him to be a good person himself, and if he can turn into a better person in life than me, then I hope he does, actually. I don't want him to be as screwed up as I am.

As this case illustrates, obtaining the parent's commitment to a nonviolent approach requires that the therapist search for a way in which such a commitment will fit for the particular parent. Mark was locked into battle with Helen, and part of his issue with her was that, since their marriage, she had been influenced by her peer group to change many of her ideas and values concerning child rearing. Mark felt put down by her attempts to change him, and the issue of "to smack" or "not to smack" became the focal point for his assertion of the old values and her assertion of the new. Mark refused to commit himself to stopping hitting the children until the therapist hit upon a way that Mark could save face while doing so. Mark would not stop hitting the children because Helen's friends said so, but would do so because he, himself, decided that he did not want his child to become aggressive like he had become. He wanted his son to have a chance to become a better person. Instead of physical discipline being a means to this end of creating a better person, a commitment to nonviolent means of discipline became one important step.

MAKING APOLOGIES PART OF THE DISCOURSE

The second area for therapy to address is the ability of family members to exit from destructive escalations by being able to acknowledge wrongdoing and by apologizing.

Sooner or later, a stage may be reached in therapy at which apology and reparation are necessary and important. Apologies acknowledge the harm done intentionally or unknowingly to the other person and, when honestly and openly undertaken, can break the hubris that underlies the cycles of exploitation and resistance characterizing family relationships.

Very often, individuals enter therapy unaware of why they have behaved destructively or with an account of their behavior that is superficial and defensive. It is through tracking the genealogy of relationships and uncovering the hidden account that the "why" of someone's behavior takes on greater authenticity and meaning. To be more than simply conceding to the therapist's demands that a person "take responsibility," and to be experienced as genuine by both the giver and receiver of the apology, an apology must come after the person comes to some understanding of why he or she committed the act and the effects of his or her behavior on others. Given the nature of hidden accounts, very often, people have only a partial understanding of *why*. If they are required by therapists to take responsibility prior to actually understanding their own behavior, the relationship with the therapist may replicate a pattern of dominance and submission that has characterized the family relationships. In this approach, the *why* of one's own behavior is constructed through the genealogical method as described in previous chapters.

The individuals in families in which physical or sexual abuse occurs are not very good at the sort of open self-confrontation and vulnerability entailed in making such an apology. It is not part of their culture. It is the therapist's responsibility, therefore, to both track the genealogy of relationships and ensure that leverage is great enough that the parents will be in agreement with the efforts of the therapist to set the stage where genuine apology can occur. The therapist is not simply interested in a particular person apologizing for a particular behavior (although a particular focus must be taken), but rather, in changing the family's discourse into one that has the possibility of self-disclosure, vulnerability, and apology.

The need for apology is most apparent in cases of sexual assault. An apology from a father who has been sexually abusive draws a clear line between past and future behavior (he undertakes never to sexualize his relationships with his children again), locates the responsibility for the abuse squarely on his shoulders, and enables him to demonstrate a one-down position in relation to his wife and children.

In cases of sexual abuse, all of this is necessary if the relationship between the father and the victim is to ever heal, as well as for ensuring the father's commitment to maintaining a new behavior pattern. The child who has been coerced into sexual assault through bribes, threats, and secrecy must also be helped to work through the legacy of guilt and misplaced responsibility (in separate sessions or separate therapy), a task that is greatly facilitated by the father apologizing and taking responsibility for the abuse.

Genuine remorse and apology from a father for sexual abuse may be difficult to obtain in the beginning of therapy, even when the hidden account relating to the father's perception of unfairness in the current family appears to have been addressed. Men may deny or minimize the consequences to their children of sexual abuse. This is, in part, because of the discourse of masculinity, which, as in the case of Arthur Dale, defines anything other than intercourse as not "real sex." The other reason, however, is that a proportion of these men were themselves sexually victimized as children. When they first enter therapy, they are disconnected from the painful feelings associated with their own abuse and, therefore, have little empathy for their victims. This constitutes another level of hidden account that must be brought back into experience before they are able to identify with the effect they have had on their victims and, therefore, make a genuine apology.

In the following excerpt from the therapy of the Orczy family, the therapist had prepared the ground for the family meeting during which the father, John, was to apologize to his daughters and take responsibility for the sexual abuse he had perpetrated over several years. In sessions prior to this, therapy had explored the story of the abuse and the genealogy of relationships (see Chapter 9). By talking for the first time about the abuse he had suffered at the hands of his brother, John began to reidentify with the fear and trauma he had experienced as a child and, in doing so, identified with the fear and trauma his daughters must have experienced. At this point, we discussed with him the possibility of arranging a family session in which he could apologize to his daughters, and he rehearsed with the therapist what he wanted to say. John's daughters were similarly prepared for this meeting through several sessions that were held with the two of them alone, and with their mother.

After exploring the changes in the family since the disclosure of the abuse, the therapist provided an opening for the father to apologize to his daughters:

THERAPIST: Take your time here to talk to them about some of the things you have been thinking about.

JOHN: (*to daughter, Sandy*) You know, when I confessed that time, I felt bad because I knew, I knew for a long time why you were getting into trouble. Did you know why you were acting up, Sandy?

SANDY: No.

JOHN: Well, I knew. Something inside me knew, but I was scared, 'cause I didn't know if I would get charged. But I still cared. I was scared, and I really cared for you. The things I done to you were sort of an impulse that I felt like I couldn't control, but I didn't want to do it to you. I knew I'd done wrong, and I just couldn't face up to people. So I wanted to be selfish and commit suicide and get it over with. I didn't want to have to go to court and face up to the therapist and tell people what I'd done, because I was gutless. But you inspired me. You stuck by me, both of you. I knew we were going to have to go to therapy. I just felt so bad, I knew we had to do something. (*turning to therapist*) It's all I can sort of say.

THERAPIST: John, sometimes when this happens, at some level, the girls blame themselves. Can you talk to them about who is responsible?

JOHN: You might have thought at the time that you were being disloyal to Mom because of what I'd done to you, but then you thought that if you told Mom, you were going to be disloyal to me, isn't that right?

SANDY: Yes (*nods*).

JEAN: Yeah.

JOHN: You was carrying that blame because you thought you had given in to me, and you hadn't said anything. And yet it was boiling up inside of you, wasn't it?

SANDY: Yes.

JOHN: Never blame yourself. I was the one to blame. You are not to blame yourselves. You've got to think back, "I was the victim." "I had the right to say no, but I couldn't," because, because you trusted me, didn't you? You looked to me for protection, and I failed you. I didn't protect you. I was supposed to protect you against people from molesting you, and I didn't do that. I molested you. I assaulted you. You have to think, "It's not my fault at all." Do you understand?

THERAPIST: It also sounds like you will understand if they go through a period of being angry with you.

JOHN: Of course. (*turning to his daughters*) I'm really sorry for everything I have done to you. I assaulted you. Nothing like this should have ever happened to you. And I hope, as time goes on, and you get older, that you will learn to forgive me. I'm not going to say, "Will you forgive me?" now, because you won't forgive me for a long while. It takes a long healing process to forgive. I can't expect to say to you, "I'm good to you now, so will you forgive me?" Because you're not, it's not true. I know that down deep there's going to be a resentment toward me.

THERAPIST: I wonder if what you need to do is to reassure them about your intentions?

JOHN: Yeah. For all my life I've had this thing inside me, this sort of pattern. Because I know what causes it now. There should *never, never* be a reoccurrence. I know in myself there never will be. I know that if I felt that way, I could go to your Mom and I could discuss it, about the way I feel. Because, you know, before, I couldn't discuss it, how I felt with anybody, and now I can discuss with Mom about how I feel, and I could tell the therapist if I felt like I was going back. I would know it in myself. And for myself, I don't want to let myself down. I don't want to let you down. I want us to be happy.

This segment of interview illustrates the context for an apology that has been structured and rehearsed. The daughters do not, and are not asked to, interact further with their father concerning his apology. He is not asking for and cannot be expected, at this stage, to receive forgiveness. Up to this point, the father and mother have been seen separately from the daughters. The apology marks the beginning point and sets the stage for work with the family as a whole.

The following case example is different. This session was not planned, the apology was not rehearsed, and the child, rather than the parent, first initiates apologizing. This segment of the interview was drawn from the latter part of the interview with the Travis family, first introduced in Chapter 9.

Sally Travis had beaten Allison, 10, after Allison had been stealing money from her purse over a period of time. In the earlier part of the interview, it became apparent that Allison had felt excluded from the close relationship her older sister had with her mother. The mother's apparent rejection of Allison was traced back to an incident in which Allison had deliberately pushed her sister over while rollerskating, causing her to be cut and bruised. Sally, the mother, maintained that beating Allison was a parent's right, an acceptable act, a last-ditch attempt to get through to Allison and stop her from stealing. Sally would not feel remorse for her actions until Allison showed some contrition. Allison would not show contrition until her position had been understood and, we believed, that by the middle of this interview, the unfairness of her exclusion and rejection was very clear. It had also become apparent during the interview that Allison was much shyer than her sister, Susan, had fewer friends, and found it difficult to talk to people. Having had a brief discussion with Allison about what it is like to be shy and have few friends, Allison brightened up and sat up straight in her chair.

THERAPIST: I had an older sister, too. And sometimes I was quite jealous of her. And she was much more outgoing, too. It must be hard for you when you don't even have your sister to be a friend with. How long do you think it will take before your sister will forgive you for pushing her over?

ALLISON: A long time.

THERAPIST: A year? Ten years? Will she be an 80-year-old lady before she forgives you? Will she be walking up to you when she's, say, 80 (*mimicking an older voice*), "Allison I forgive you"?

ALLISON: (*Smiles and shrugs.*)

THERAPIST: (*to mother*) What do you think?

MOTHER: (*visibly softening*) Not very long. Susan is very forgiving.

THERAPIST: Do you think that Susan knows how much Allison suffers==

MOTHER: ==No. . . . I don't think that she sees what's inside Allison. I don't think Susan sits back and has a look at the situation.

THERAPIST: So, when you think about how long it will take for her to forgive her, what do you think? Less than 80 years? Would you imagine it would be a long time or a short time? Months, years, weeks?

MOTHER: Weeks.

THERAPIST: Do you think that Allison would have to do anything for Susan to forgive her?

MOTHER: Yes, I do. I think Allison would have to show Susan that she feels something for Susan, and once she showed her that, Susan would forget it completely, drop it.

THERAPIST: Has Allison ever apologized to Susan for it?

MOTHER: No.

THERAPIST: Why is that? Do you think she's too proud?

MOTHER: Yes.

THERAPIST: So who's the proudest between the two of them? Who's the one who's most proud, so that they could never say to the other one, "Listen, I still want to be friends with you"?

MOTHER: I mean, I couldn't imagine Susan doing something like that in the first place. I think when Allison does things, she's sorry herself, but she find it extremely difficult. She feels it inside (*gesturing to her heart*), but it ties her up in knots. But to get that out in words (*gesturing from her mouth outward*), but to get that out, is hard.

THERAPIST: (*to Allison*) Do you think your mom is understanding you right there?

ALLISON: Yes.

The mother's tone and posture have changed by this stage. Rather than the sullen, withdrawn presentation at the beginning of the interview, she has taken the position of expert with her children and is perceptive and articulate. She seemed softer, warmer. Much of what she attributed to Susan also described how she, herself, felt and reacted. She was hurt and rejected by Allison's rejection of her and too proud to make a first move toward Allison. And yet her distance from Allison covered over a deeper attachment and longing to be close to her, which could emerge if some contact could be made.

THERAPIST: Is your mom reading you right? (*Allison nods.*) How do you feel about what happened with the rollerskates?

ALLISON: (*very seriously and intently*) Sorry.

THERAPIST: Have you ever told your sister?

ALLISON: (*shaking her head*) No.

THERAPIST: How do you think she would react if you did?

ALLISON: (*shaking her head*) I don't know.

THERAPIST: Do you think she would accept it, or do you think she would push it away?

At this stage, Susan distracted herself from the intensity of this moment by picking at some recent scabs on her feet. This had the effect of restoring the mother's attention to her as blood oozed under the scab, and the mother told her not to pick at it. The session was interrupted as I searched for tissues to deal with the scab.

I asked Allison, and then after that, Susan, how each of them thought the other would respond if Allison approached Susan. Both replied, "I don't know." Allison look sad, whereas, Susan looked irritated and picked more at the scab. Susan, I expected, was unwilling to be easily won over, given that this might mean the loss of her privileged position with her mother.

THERAPIST: And do you think you would accept it and forgive her, or do you think you wouldn't?

SUSAN: Not really . . . 'cause I haven't ever apologized to anyone. I mean, I haven't even said it's all right, it's OK to anyone.

THERAPIST: (*to mother*) Do you think that's a good thing or a bad thing?

MOTHER: I think that's a bad thing!

THERAPIST: Who do you think she's getting that from?

MOTHER: I don't know (*stiffening slightly in her chair*).

THERAPIST: Do you think she might be getting it from some of the kids at school?

MOTHER: It's possible that she could be getting it from school. I don't know who she's doing this with at school, but she's definitely not getting it from me.

THERAPIST: No, it doesn't seem to be your view.

MOTHER: No.

The implication that Susan was supported in this position by her mother was hinted at and then avoided as a way of pointing out the problem while keeping the mother's alliance. Sally is challenged to ensure that Allison's apology would be accepted by Susan and, ultimately, by herself.

THERAPIST: Who do you think would be best at helping her get her thoughts straightened out about it?

MOTHER: (*after pausing for a long while*) Well, probably me.

THERAPIST: Do you think so? Does she listen to you?

MOTHER: Susan listens to me, yeah.

THERAPIST: So she may be proud and tough, but she's also open.

THERAPIST: (*to Susan*) Do you think your sister has pulled away from your mom, as well as away from you?

SUSAN: Nah.

THERAPIST: (*to Allison, who is now looking away*) Do you think that out of what's happened, you've pulled away from your mom as well as from your sister?

ALLISON: What does that mean?

THERAPIST: It means that you kind of pull in so that you don't talk to them (*gesturing hands pulled in toward the heart and closed in*).

ALLISON: (*nodding*) Yeah.

THERAPIST: So you think that has happened? With your mom, or with your sister, or with both?

ALLISON: (*nodding and turning away*) I don't know.

THERAPIST: (*to mother*) What do you think?

MOTHER: I think with both.

THERAPIST: Do you think that's because she's been feeling so bad about what's happened, or==

MOTHER: ==Yeah, I do. I think because of the money incident, and as it continued, she felt really bad about that. She's been given a few months to think about what she's done. And because of that, she's felt rather shut off from me (*closing her arms over her heart and pulling inward, as I had done previously*), and because of the rollerskating incident and feeling bad about that, and not apologizing to Susan for doing it, and feeling hurt inside, she withdrew.

Sally's increasing understanding and empathy was evident. Her description of Susan's reaction, "Susan didn't step back out of the situation to look at it," also seemed to be a reference to her own reaction. She had not been able to see Allison's behavior as it evolved through the incident at school, with the rollerskates, and the rejection from Susan. By this stage, Allison had become less the "bad child." In fact, the negative aspects of Susan's behavior have been highlighted: her lack of empathy, her pride, her unwillingness to resolve the situation. Thus, the extreme complementarity or splitting between the two children has decreased. Instead of Allison, "the bad child," the punctuation is reversed: Allison was being victimized by Susan's unwillingness to forgive Allison's past mistakes. Thus, Susan needed help from her mother to overcome this problem and her pride.

THERAPIST: (*to mother*) Has Allison apologized to you for the money incident?

MOTHER: No.

THERAPIST: How do you think she does feel about that? (*Allison covers her face with her hand and looks away.*)

MOTHER: Well, I feel she must feel bad about it.

THERAPIST: (*to Allison*) Is that right?

ALLISON: (*Nods sadly or in shame.*)

THERAPIST: And you feel sorry about it, but you haven't ever told your mom that? (*Allison nods.*) How do you think your mom would respond if you were to tell her?

ALLISON: (*shaking her head*) I don't know.

By allowing her to reflect upon how she would respond to the questioning prepared the mother to respond differently to Allison. I stood up and took Allison's hand, leading her to the empty chair beside her mother. I pulled my chair closer to Allison and leaned forward, talking softly to her.

THERAPIST: Let's try it out and see what she says, OK? Tell your mom how you feel about taking the money.

ALLISON: (*turning to her mother and speaking softly*) I feel sad.

MOTHER: Do you?

ALLISON: Yes.

MOTHER: I don't have to sleep with my purse underneath my pillow any more?

ALLISON: (*shaking her head*) No.

Sally reached over and took Allison's hand, squeezing it. Both of them smiled through their tears. As Sally squeezed Allison's hand harder, Allison laughed, saying, "Ow!"

MOTHER: And I *do* forgive you for doing it. OK?

I expected that at that point Sally would have swept Allison into her arms. But instead, she sat motionless, only her dewy eyes portraying her deeper feeling. I had to facilitate in some way the next step.

THERAPIST: Who needs the hug the most, the mom or the daughter?

Allison jumped out of her seat and into her mothers's arms. Sally held her, rocking her gently back and forth and whispered, "I'm sorry, I love you." Allison whispered, "I love you, too." I sat silently for 5 minutes as they talked. Susan sat silently in the other chair beside her mother, picking at her scabs. Allison eventually climbed off her mother's lap, both of them joking about how quickly she was growing up. Sally wiped the tears from her face.

I gestured for Allison to sit down again in the chair. I looked toward her mother. Our postures mirrored each other—both of us had one hand resting on the side of our faces, thoughtfully.

THERAPIST: I wonder (*long pause*), I wonder whether Allison is mature enough inside herself to say that she is sorry to her sister, even though her sister at this stage is too proud and, in a sense, too immature to be able to accept it.

MOTHER: I think she could do that.

THERAPIST: Do you think she is mature enough to do that?

MOTHER: Well, she's growing up, isn't she. She's nearly 10.

THERAPIST: (*to Allison*) What do you think?

ALLISON: What does that mean? I don't know.

THERAPIST: "Mature" means, like, in a way you're grown up, become responsible in that way. Do you think that you're, in a way, grown up enough to tell your sister that you're sorry, even though she's not grown up enough right now to be able to accept it?

ALLISON: I think I'm grown up enough.

I pulled a chair closer to Susan's chair, and Allison moved into it. "Susan," I said, "your sister's got something to tell you." Allison spoke for herself immediately:

ALLISON: I'm sorry that I pushed you off the rollerskates.

Susan looked away from Allison with both hands on the top of her head, saying nothing. Finally she turned to her mother and said, "I don't know what to say."

THERAPIST: (*to Allison*) Do you want to be friends again with her?

ALLISON: (*Nods and then whispers to Susan.*) I want to be friends again.

We all sat in silence for a long minute. Sally and I stared down to the ground, trying not to cue Susan. Susan, I suspect, was somewhat torn. She felt the pressure to give a "mature" response, knowing that this was the only way that she could maintain her status. On the other hand, to do so would free Allison from being the "bad girl" and put Susan in the position of losing her special privilege as the "good girl."

THERAPIST: (*to Allison*) You've done very well. I think you're more like, at least, 12. (*Allison smiles.*) It's hard when you've hurt feelings and you're a shy person. It's hard to tell people when you're hurt. (*Allison nods.*)

MOTHER: (*to Allison*) How do you feel about the rumors you spread about Susan? . . . How do you feel about the bad things you said at school? Losing your sister's friends and your brother's friends?

ALLISON: I feel sad about that.

MOTHER: (*to therapist*) That could be part of what's keeping Susan apart.

THERAPIST: I see.

THERAPIST: (*to Allison*) Do you want to apologize to her about that, too?

ALLISON: (*nodding*) I'm sorry about the things that I said about you at school.

SUSAN: It doesn't matter. They'll all back, because I told them the truth.

THERAPIST: Does that mean you've forgiven her for that?

SUSAN: For that, yeah.

THERAPIST: Tell her, so that she knows it.

SUSAN: That's OK. I apologize, too. OK?

At this point, the two sisters broke into an animated discussion concerning two of their friends. They had connected. They were friends again. I turned to Sally and arranged the next appointment.

This session and the apologies that were a part of it, were a breakthrough for the family in finding a way out of the escalation of power and resistance in which they had been caught. From this session grew the motivation of both Allison and her mother, as well as Allison's sibling, to reconnect and reestablish their relationships. On her own accord, Sally arranged for each child to have a special time with her once each week, and sibling rivalry decreased. Allison and Susan became good friends once again. In talking with Allison during later sessions, Sally was able to reach through what she called Allison's "wall," and later, "bubble." Allison's withdrawal from her and subsequent "wall," Sally discovered, had at its core that Allison felt that she was "bad" inside and unworthy of her mother's love. Sally convinced her otherwise. Sally also established a relationship with a caring man. Commenting on how different she felt in this relationship, Sally described how her own "bubble" had disappeared through helping Allison with hers.

RESOLVING CONFLICTS: COMMITMENT TO FAIRNESS AND EQUITY

The third aspect of an ethical base for relating is for family members to become committed to fairness and equity in their relationships with others.

As described in Chapter 5, the inability to resolve relationship conflicts in a manner that feels fair to those concerned contributes to an escalation of behaviors ultimately leading to a parent choosing physical or sexual abuse as an option. It is important, therefore, that, in addition to developing a commitment to respect and nonviolence and the ability to apologize and accept apologies, parents develop a willingness to address relationship conflicts and see that important issues are resolved fairly. Some of these will be issues or injustices that contributed to the abusive parent's feelings of resentment and exclusion. Others will have arisen in response to the secrecy and coalitions that were an inevitable part of the abusive context, and still others will be issues that remain unfinished from family of origin experiences. In the following sections we provide case examples of these types of relationship issues.

Issues Contributing to the Abuse

In terms of diffusing the abusive parent's desire to hurt and the motivation for further abuse, it is important to resolve relationship conflicts that fed the abusive parent's sense of injustice and contributed to their anger and resentment.

The situation of the Nicolopoulos family, in which George had sexually assaulted his 16-year-old daughter, provides a good example of such issues. This case demonstrates one of the situations where relationship questions alone were not sufficient to change an unfair situation. The major change in relationships, instead, happened after the mother was coerced, through the therapist's leverage, to adopt a different position.

Recall that Fatima Nicolopoulos had felt pressured into marrying George when she became pregnant. Her father had allowed the marriage on the condition that Fatima and any children of the marriage have no contact with George's family. The couple had conflicted over the years as to whether the children should ever meet George's parents. Fatima had remained firm, however, and the children, now in their teens, had never met George's parents or their aunts and uncles, despite living in the same city. George felt rejected by his wife and, ultimately, by his children as they grew older and formed a coalition against him. He felt on the emotional periphery of both his own family and his family of origin. His resistance to this was to become increasingly dominating and controlling, to which, in response, his wife and children banded together against him, increasing his feelings of exclusion. Both Fatima and the children felt dominated and controlled.

Therapy with this family initially focused on the issues as defined by the mother and children: the abuse, George's autocratic control, and the lack of openness and communication between George and other family members. Changes in George's behavior were facilitated by the leverage inherent in George's desire to return home. As family relationships changed, George again raised the issue of the children never having met their paternal grandparents. He expressed his grief about the children not seeing their grandparents, and his anger with his wife about what he believed to be an unfair situation. This significant and long-standing issue had contributed to George's feelings of rejection and unfairness.

Fatima, however, appeared to be unmoved by George's pleas and refused to budge from her position of forbidding any contact between the children and grandparents, despite our attempts during the session to have her reconsider. Seeing her individually, we told her that the children would not be safe with George until this issue was resolved fairly. If he were to return home before then, we would perceive their daughter to be at risk of further abuse, and we would be obligated to notify the Department. Knowing that Fatima was very interested in George returning home as soon as possible, we used the leverage inherent in this situation to encourage Fatima to adopt a fair position in relation to this issue. During this meeting, Fatima held steadfast and refused to change her position. We perceived Fatima as unwilling to lose her hold over George in the one area where she held any significant power. Given his mistreatment of their daughter and of Fatima, herself, we could understand her need to do so. However, the requirement that George sacrifice his relationship with his family was unfair. Until he could have a relationship with both his wife and children, and his own family, we did not expect that he would maintain his willingness to commit himself to behaving fairly in his relationships with others.

Over the next 2 weeks, however, Fatima reconsidered and changed her mind. In the following session, George wept openly as he described the children's first meeting with their grandparents, aunts, and uncles. With this issue resolved between the couple, George's approach to his wife and children softened. His efforts at developing a more open and egalitarian relationship with them no longer represented a "compromise" but, rather, a genuine shift in how he wished to relate to them.

Issues of Unfairness Arising as a Result of the Abuse

In working with the legacy of relationships shattered by abuse, it is important to address relationship conflicts that arise as a direct effect of the abuse. Being excluded from relationships, feeling favored or rejected are all intensified when abuse has occurred. When the abuse has stopped and therapy has addressed the abuse and issues fueling the abuse, other more apparently everyday issues will present, which, when explored, can still be seen to have their origins in the relationships created through the abuse.

A few months into therapy with the Orczy family, and during a whole family session, Leanne, age 17, reported that she and Sandy, 16, had argued bitterly when Leanne discovered that Sandy had "borrowed" several of her music tapes. Leanne complained that Sandy often went into her room and took things without asking. When we inquired about relationships between the siblings, and between the daughters and their parents, Sandy revealed feeling alienated in the family and excluded from a close relationship with her siblings. It became clear during the session that Sandy's alienation in the family had been an effect of the abuse. Feeling bad about herself, she had withdrawn from her mother and become jealous of her sister's apparent closeness to the mother. Her more distant relationship to her mother had also made her an easier target for victimization.

THERAPIST: (*to John*) How do you see the relationship between Leanne and her mom compared to the relationship between Sandy and her mom?

JOHN: Sandy's jealous. I think it's always been that way with Sandy since she was a little child, that she sort of got pushed out of the way a bit. She's very sensitive, always has been. I think that she wanted to be sort of part of the group, but she felt she wasn't accepted. Because we had adopted her, and she had lost her own mother. I think that by taking things, she feels like she's got part of what they have.

THERAPIST: (*to Leanne*) What do you think Sandy would be jealous of in your relationship with your mom?

Leanne: Maybe because we talk a lot.

Leanne described herself as temperamentally more similar to her mother, both of them very different from Sandy's volatility. When they were younger, Leanne said she resented Sandy because she believed that Sandy manipulated their mother and "tried to get away with things." When the therapist inquired about the relationship between the two sisters, Sandy replied that she believed that Leanne felt "0 out of 100" close to her. Saying this, she began to cry, and Leanne, in turn, appeared to soften. Leanne responded by saying that she felt about "60" in terms of closeness to Sandy but that she wanted to feel much closer. The therapist turned to the mother, Rita:

THERAPIST: Before therapy, how close do you think that Sandy felt to you compared to what Leanne felt to you?

RITA: Well, I'd say Sandy was about 50%, and Leanne would probably be about 70%.

THERAPIST: And what would you say it is now?

RITA: Well, I'd say that Sandy is probably up to about 70%, but now Leanne would be higher, too, so she might be 80%.

THERAPIST: And how do you see it, Sandy?

SANDY: I'm getting closer to Mom now than I was before. And Leanne's getting closer now to Mom, too, because they're talking more.

THERAPIST: Do you think that you could ever get as close to your mom as what Leanne is? Is that a possibility or not?

SANDY: Maybe not quite as close, but close enough.

RITA: From my part, definitely, yes. I'm working on it. I'm determined to get her just as close. It does take some doing. I want it very much.

In asking Rita about the relationship between each daughter and their father, we were told that although both relationships had improved, Sandy still appeared to "hold back a little more." Rita attributed this difference to John's preferential treatment of Leanne in the past, leaving Sandy to think that "John loved Leanne much more, very much more." To this, Sandy agreed:

THERAPIST: You must have felt very lost and alone in terms of your relationship with your dad, and also with your mom and Leanne.

SANDY: Yes (*continuing to cry intermittently in the session, wiping her tears with tissues*).

THERAPIST: Sandy, I wonder if part of what was going on is that during the time that you were being abused, you didn't know that your sister was also being abused. You thought at the time that it was only you.

SANDY: Yeah, I thought that Dad wasn't interfering with Leanne. I thought it was just me, and that's why I thought that Dad hated me, and that he loved those three. I thought he could never love me as much as he loves Leanne.

Because of her adoption, Sandy said, she had always felt excluded from the relationships with her older sister and brother. For many years, she believed she was the only one who was being assaulted by her father and that this indicated her father's preference for her older sister who was the "real daughter," while Sandy remained the "adopted daughter." The secret of the abuse had separated and alienated them.

THERAPIST: Because you thought that you were the only one in the family that he was hurting. You thought that you were alone.

SANDY: Before, we just didn't share our feelings much. And I thought that they didn't love me. And I thought Mom didn't love me because she wasn't protecting me, and Leanne, 'cause I couldn't talk to her, and Jason and Daryl because they liked each other the best, and Dad, because of what he was doing to me.

THERAPIST: You felt pretty alone. I'm surprised you were only stealing music tapes!

SANDY: (*Laughs.*)

JOHN: Can I just add something to all that? It used to be that one month, I would love Leanne more than Sandy. And the next month. I would love Sandy more than Leanne. It would go up and down.

THERAPIST: And I guess that would add to their rivalry. How much do you think that Sandy now thinks that you love her in a true sort of fatherly, healthy way?

JOHN: I think she's gone up to about 3 or 4 out of 10. She's still not certain.

THERAPIST: And before?

JOHN: Before it would have been about 1. But she's always been quite loving. She would come up and hug me. She does that even more now, and I respect her for that.

THERAPIST: So somehow this feeling of being left out has not killed the love inside her. And how do you think your dad is reading you, Sandy?

SANDY: Yeah, I think it would be about 3 or 4.

THERAPIST: How much do you think that *he thinks* that he loves you?

SANDY: (*pause*) I don't know. Probably about 4.

THERAPIST: (*to John*) And what would you say?

JOHN: No, higher, about 7ish.

THERAPIST: So she's a bit low on her ratings! (*Sandy and her father laugh.*) She's not receiving the message very clearly.

JOHN: Yeah, I do love her, and I wouldn't like to see anything happen to her.

This session highlighted the painful position in which Sandy found herself and provided her with the opportunity to clarify her misperceptions of how others valued her. Subsequent to this session and over the next several months, Sandy became much closer to her sister, Leanne, and to both of her parents. When John maintained the changes in his behavior and attitudes over the next several months, Sandy became more trusting of him, and the two had frequent open and spontaneous conversations.

Family-of-Origin Issues

Finally, some of the unresolved relationship issues that fuel current relationship patterns are situated in past relationships with family of origin. In the situation of John Orczy, for example, two issues that featured highly were the loss of his great aunt when he was very young and the sexual assault by his brother when he was 8 years old. The loss of his great aunt was significant in that she had been a loving caretaker of him for a year, until he was 3 years old. Following her death he was frequently neglected by his parents. After John had made significant changes in his own family, we approached dealing with these issues with him. One session was spent focused on his relationship with his great aunt. John described feeling rejected and abandoned by her through her death and also guilty that he had never said good-bye. He was able to reestablish contact with his hidden and unresolved grief and received care and support from his wife.

A session was later arranged with his own parents, now aged in their 70s and 80s. John's parents were not the people they had been during John's childhood. Both were frail and hard of hearing, and it was hard to imagine John's father as a strong and violent man. During this session, John talked about the loss of his great aunt and the changes in family relationships that followed. His parents spoke about the financial hardship they had suffered and the need for his mother to go out to work. His mother described how she had become very depressed following the death of the great aunt, who had been like a mother to her, and how this in some way contributed to her neglect of him.

After starting therapy, John had told his parents about having sexually abused his daughters. He had never, however, told them of having been assaulted by his brother during his own childhood. During this session, he revealed this to them, describing how the assault had affected him, and how he feared ever telling his father because of his father's violence. His parents listened intently and recalled as much as possible of the situation for them at the time. John's mother revealed that she, herself, had been sexually "interfered with" by her own father, and that she believed that this had in some way affected her ability to protect him. Although this session was important to John, it did not have the impact of a subsequent session, where John spoke with the brother who had abused him.

John had never discussed or confronted his brother, Peter, about having abused him. Unlike John's parents, Peter had never immigrated to Australia, and he and John had had little contact over the years. When Peter arrived for a holiday during the course of therapy, John had the opportunity to talk to him for the first time in 15 years. John invited him to a therapy session, explaining that he needed help for "a problem of violence." He told Peter that he was trying to recall aspects of his childhood and needed Peter's help.

The following is an excerpt from the session in which John confronted his brother regarding the abuse. Prior to this session, we had explored with John what he wished to discuss with Peter and how he would do so. In beginning the session, the therapist spent some time connecting with Peter and then explored with the brothers their recollections of their relationship as children. John described Peter as good to him in many ways, taking him to the pictures and spending time with him. He recalled, however, that Peter had a very violent temper, describing the day Peter had thrown a chair through the front window.

JOHN: He was pretty cruel at times.

THERAPIST: In what way?

JOHN: He used to tie me up and use me for target practice. He would throw stuff at me.

PETER: (*laughs*) Oh, yeah, apples and stuff.

JOHN: He sexually assaulted me.

PETER: Huh?

JOHN: You sexually assaulted me==

PETER: ==Hold on, how do you mean?

JOHN: ==You forced me to have oral sex with you, Peter.

PETER: Ah (*places his hand to his head*), that's right. I was trying to==

JOHN: ==OK, put it this way, Peter, I'm not holding resentment over it, but I always have flashbacks on that. Actually, I forgot a lot until I started to come into puberty myself. I never hated you for it. I sort of looked at it this way, I sort of put down a lot to our background.

PETER: Yeah.

JOHN: I've done things to the girls because of the anger, the anger in me, because you got angry with me sometimes and it was sexual, so it came out that way. Ah, I'm not holding you to blame, I'm not saying you're to blame, but what it is, it is like a chain of events. I wondered sometimes, because of the way that Dad belted you around, it might have affected you sexually. Because I can remember you, you was about 12, and I used to feel sorry for you, 'cause you used to wear glasses and used to look very vague. I can still see how you looked, now. But I always had that feeling that you got pushed around. That's why I never went to Mom or Dad, or said anything to them. 'Cause I knew they'd crack up on you.

PETER: It was only a couple of times or something.

JOHN: It was three or four times. That's irrelevant. After that I used to say "no" and that was it. But you did something to me. You wanted me to have oral sex with you and you did something. I don't know what happened that day, but you were very angry. I'll sort of go ahead and see if you can remember.

PETER: Yes.

JOHN: I'm not digging out the past, I'm==

PETER: ==No, no, go ahead. These were war years.

JOHN: What happened there was you wanted me to have oral sex with you and I said, "No," and you used to bribe me. But one day, I think what stuck in my mind more than anything was you started smashing me across the face.

PETER: Did I?

JOHN: And the old man heard it. He was way down in the garden, and he came running up. And I was worried. I knew that would be Dad's shining chance to really eliminate you. He would have really beaten you bad, I reckon. But I wouldn't talk. But from that day onwards, something changed in me.

The duration of the session was spent exploring the family relationships at the time Peter had assaulted John. Peter described the intimidation he felt from his own father and the threat that John, who was the younger and preferred son, posed to him. He had felt angry and excluded. In leaving the room at the end of this session, John proclaimed that something profound had changed inside him.

Although John Orczy's assault by his brother more than 30 years ago and George Nicolopoulos's resigned despair about his children not being allowed to see his parents were very different issues, one 30 years old and one current, both situations involved the abusive parent feeling unjustly treated. By taking these experiences seriously and assisting the parent in resolving and achieving some sense of justice, these fathers were able to release their attachment to issues that fueled their own unjust and unfair treatment of others.

By taking seriously the hurt and rejection experienced by both the abusive parent and other family members, the therapist facilitates the family in creating a different ideal for relationships. This ideal is one in which feelings of abandonment and rejection are openly acknowledged and worked through, rather than acted out in retribution, an ideal in which oppression and control of others is rejected in favor of respect and caring.

Conclusion

I wrote this book as a protest against the dominant professional discourses concerning child abuse. In particular, I wanted to demonstrate that child abuse is not simply the outcome of individual or family pathology, but rather, the inevitable outcome of an individual's position within gender and class contexts, as well as a particular genealogy of relationships. The disease discourse of child abuse fails to consider the meaning and impact of individuals' positions and the circumstances under which they become "clients." The result of this failing is that the perpetrators of child abuse become genderless "parents," and classless and stageless "families." The pathologizing of parents and families by therapists and other "social helpers" constructs a "problem," a "dysfunction," that, seen differently, is a conflict and struggle—socially between classes, clinically between professionals and parents, and interfamilially between genders and generations.

The lack of attention given to gender obscures the fact that the vast majority of clients of child protection services are women, even when they are not the alleged abusers. A question never raised within the disease discourse is the degree to which women are coerced into subordinate relationships with professionals, relationships that replicate the patriarchal arrangement in which many women are caught or from which they are fleeing. Also never examined is the unwillingness or inability of professionals to successfully engage and work with men.

I have also sought to demonstrate that resistance to intervention should not simply be explained as reflecting the parents' "pathology." Gender and class location, life stage, and the parents' particular situation largely account for their struggles for autonomy or desperation for help. These contexts construct the states of mind from which professional intervention is construed as controlling, caring, or dismissing. Child abuse emerges from within the very strains, contradictions, and conflicts of

233

interest inherent in gender relations and family life, and the parents'
openness to professionals depends very much on the professionals' timing
and location.

The parents' "resistance" to therapy is also intimately connected to
the impact of involuntary referral to both the CP Department and to
therapy. The approach taken in this book, however, demonstrates that
even when referral to therapy is involuntary, "resistance" need not be an
inevitable outcome. When leverage is in place and parents stand to gain
from attending therapy, when parents are given some element of choice,
and when they are given the opportunity to tell their story, the face of
"resistance" changes considerably.

This book has taken the position that therapy must in some way
address the values and premises that support abusive and authoritarian
practices. Although intervention by the CP Department may stop abuse
or punish the offender, in most cases it does not facilitate a behavioral or
attitudinal change in the abuser that might be termed "therapeutic."
Confrontation by a CP Worker may be effective in setting limits on
parents' behavior, conveying that they have breached acceptable standards. An intervention of this sort utilizes the leverage inherent in CP
Workers' greater power and authority, and fits well within abusive parents'
constructions of the world. It nevertheless displays a force that may serve
to reinforce the very premises on which an abusive parent's behavior is
based. Unless intervention can challenge these premises and change the
values underlying abusive behaviors, it is likely that these parents will use
verbal abuse and intimidation even if they restrain themselves from
physically striking out.

If, as a society, we do wish to impose a particular discourse concerning
parent–child relationships, it may be more effective to promote change
on a larger scale rather than simply ordering to therapy those parents who
represent the extreme end of the continuum. The media, for example,
could promote alternative views of masculinity and femininity, and different conceptions of heterosexual and parent–child relationships. Schools
could create child care experiences for both boys and girls, and provide a
framework for the development of relationship values and skills. Interventions of this order would be preventive rather than after the fact, and
would reach a wider section of the population.

The most obvious reason that intervention on this scale is not
attempted is financial and this, in essence, is a question of political
priorities. A less obvious reason is that there would likely be large-scale
opposition to what could be seen as an overt manipulation of values and
the presumption that one group has the authority to tell others how to
live and relate. The marketing of a discourse that calls into question
authoritarian practices and places at its center the experiential reality of

the other would also force us to examine more closely the treatment of children in schools and day-care centers, the oppression of men and women in the workplace, exploitation of women's labor, and violence perpetrated against women in the home. In other words, although society as a whole is responsible for promoting the very practices that underpin the behavior of parents who abuse, it is parents who are found guilty, reported to "the Welfare," and sent to therapy. This confirms them as "not one of us" but, rather, our "other." We are like the fox caught in the trap, which chews off its injured leg.

Therapy becomes the carrier in which ideological tinkering may take place on a smaller scale. In accepting such a position, therapists are faced with a paradox: How can we assist parents to reconstruct their values and relationships to ones less patriarchal, less unnecessarily controlling, more interested and respectful of the other, without in the process invoking an authoritarian relationship between ourselves and the parents? How do we avoid becoming oppressive while seeking to end oppression? The contradictions of the situation emerge most profoundly with coerced or reluctant referrals to therapy, and this is one reason why therapists would rather avoid such work.

By refusing or abandoning these cases, however, we do not do the parents or their children any favor. Although parents may discontinue overt violence as a result of child protection intervention, without therapy they may nevertheless continue intimidation, authoritarian practices, and scapegoating behavior. Furthermore, when secured into the child protection system without the support of an external advocate, parents (often women on their own) are quite likely to become hopelessly entangled and further enraged as confusing and contradictory expectations of CP Workers reinforce the sense of their victimization and confirm their premises concerning relationships and power.

We must begin our relationship with these parents by offering them our concern and respect, hope of disentangling themselves from the child protection web, support in the face of what is experienced as overwhelming invasion and powerlessness, and an empathic hearing of their distress. We must make space for them to tell their story: their story of their experience with professionals, and their story of the unfolding relationships within their family.

Our position in such a framework is neither on the side of parents against the Department or the Department against the parents. Delicately unraveling the contradictory demands of the CP Department, we must transform these demands into workable objectives for parents. We must find and put into place leverage for change and, once trusted by parents to be working in the service of their deeper interests and relationships, unravel the contradictions and layers of unfairness in gender and family relationships. If, in this process, we can demonstrate respect for the experiential reality of the other and a concern for fair and equitable relationships, we reach the heart of the changes parents must make when they have been abusive.

All therapists concerned about authoritarian practices and the abuse of power need to recognize and deal with such practices whenever they are encountered. This may be in parent–child relations, marital relations, between parents and professionals, or between ourselves and our own clients. Whether we like it or not, whether we choose to recognize it or not, *we are* the power brokers.

The Research Project

T HE grounded theory presented in the first half of this book (Chapters 1 to 4) and which primarily informs the therapy project (Chapters 5 to 10) was drawn from the results of a qualitative research project I conducted from 1985 to 1991 in the State of New South Wales, Australia (MacKinnon, 1992). This appendix outlines the research method employed, describing the interview methodology, the sample, and the method of analyzing the respondents' accounts of their experiences.

The research project set out to elicit and analyze clients' accounts of professional intervention by State Child Protection authorities (at that time known as the Department of Youth and Community Services, or YACS) and public sector therapists in situations where there were allegations of child abuse.

ENLISTING THE PARTICIPANTS

The core of this research centered upon in-depth interviews with families whose children were considered to be at risk of abuse. It was also supported by in-depth interviews with therapists and frontline workers (District Officers, or D.O.s) from YACS, many of whom were involved with these families. Additionally, however, I maintained an active involvement as a participant/observer for over 4 years as a therapist working with families considered at risk of abuse, as a consultant to five teams of therapists who often worked with such cases, and as a consultant to the New South Wales. Child Protection Council that conducted interagency workshops throughout New South Wales.

Enlisting Family Members

When I began this study, I found it difficult to find parents willing to discuss their experiences with child protection intervention, a problem experienced by other researchers (Magura & Moses, 1984). Researchers generally do not have direct access to respondents. They must go through *someone* to reach the person to be interviewed. That *someone's* relationship with the respondent is therefore critical in terms of both gaining access and affecting how the researcher is likely to be perceived by the respondent.

I initially attempted to obtain participants for this study through the Department of Youth and Community Services. The red tape of YACS, however, was cumbersome, and the gatekeepers had little motivation in ensuring that clients were referred to me. Despite having official permission to interview their clients, and despite friendly discussions with several district managers, I obtained only three families directly through YACS. Because I was interested in families who had experienced both therapy and YACS, I decided to rely on other sources. I attempted to obtain subjects by using my contacts in the family therapy field by asking therapists if they had families who would be willing to talk with me. Although therapists seemed interested and reassured me of the value of my study, I initially received no referrals in this way. When I was subsequently asked by social workers and psychologists working as therapists at a public health center to supervise family therapy, I agreed to provide supervision if they could locate families interested in participating in my project. Some months later, I negotiated similar arrangements with two other centers. Once the study was under way and I began discussing aspects of it with others, I was referred cases by therapists from other centers.

In contrast to the volunteering method I had initially employed, the *quid pro quo* arrangement with the centers yielded several benefits. Interested in supervision, the therapists overcame their fears and mistrust, and were motivated to encourage families to talk to me. In order to provide the number of families required, therapists were obliged to nominate their "failures" as well as their successful cases. I interviewed not only satisfied clients but also dissatisfied ones, some who had seen therapists only once, and others who had "prematurely" dropped out of therapy dissatisfied. All but three families who were approached by therapists consented to be interviewed. Neither professionals nor families were paid for their participation.

Because the only criteria for referral to the project was that either D.O.s or therapists believed that the child had been or was at risk of being abused, the sample reflects both situations in which it was alleged that one or both parents abused the child and situations where someone outside the family was suspected of abuse. Of those parents alleged to have abused, some had identified themselves as abusive or as at risk of being abusive. Others admitted their behavior but denied that it was abusive, whereas still others simply denied the alleged behavior.

Enlisting Therapists and D.O.s

Although the initial aim of the study was not to document the accounts of therapists and D.O.s concerning their own work contexts, the need to do so became evident to me as I sought explanations for parents' accounts of professionals' behavior. My knowledge of the context of D.O.s and therapists was broadly based, drawing from my experience as a participant/observer as well as from formal interviews. From the position of therapist, I maintained ongoing contact with several D.O.s and thus had many opportunities to observe their behavior as well as my own in the management of difficult cases. As a supervisor, I maintained fortnightly contact for an average of 2 years with therapists at the three health centers that referred families to this study. Over this time, I gained a deeper understanding of the frustrations and difficulties of therapists' work, the difficulties they had in working with other agencies, and their personal struggles and feelings of inadequacy in dealing with child protection cases.

Formal interviews were conducted with 20 therapists and 8 D.O.s who had worked with the families who were being interviewed for the study. Because therapists provided many of the families for interviews, therapists were physically accessible. Many of the D.O.s of whom parents spoke had changed offices or left the Department and were thus not easily contacted.

INTERVIEW METHODOLOGY

Interviews with the 44 families were conducted during 1986 and 1987. Although most interviews were carried out in a room in the health center where the therapist worked, several occurred in the families' homes. The interviews lasted an average of 1½ hours. All except two of the interviews were taped and subsequently transcribed. Interviews were open-ended and unstructured. I began each interview by asking the parents to tell me the story of their involvement with therapists and YACS. Through the questioning process, I tracked the patterns of relationships that had developed between the family members and professionals over time. When a family had seen several professionals, I explored the differences they perceived between the professionals and how each relationship had changed over time.

Perhaps not surprisingly, the roles of researcher and therapist also merged at times. In several instances, the researcher role, free as it was from expectations of having to change the parents, at times allowed a more therapeutic encounter than the existing therapist–client relationship. Some therapists reported being less "stuck" following the research interview, and some parents reconsidered their viewpoints. It was, in fact, the success of this approach in engaging parents that was then taken up later in the therapy project.

All family members were informed of the purpose and possible outcomes of the research project. All, except one, consented to video- or audiotaping and to the interviews being used for teaching and research purposes.

THE SAMPLE

The Families

Twenty therapists referred 40 families to this study, and 4 families were referred from D.O.s. Of the 44 families, 38 were seen by at least one therapist and one D.O., 4 were seen only by D.O.s, and 2 were seen only by therapists. As is characteristic of child-at-risk cases, most families in this study had seen more than one therapist and had frequently experienced several D.O.s.

The choice of who should attend the interview was ultimately left with the parents. Some parents brought their children; others did not. Mothers constituted the majority of the respondents and were not interviewed in only four cases. Fathers were interviewed in 12 instances and children in 11. The total number of interviews was in excess of 50, as in some circumstances I interviewed children separately as well as together with their parents.

Forty-one percent were single-parent mothers (30% separated and 11% never married). In 34% of the cases, parents were in their first married or *de facto* relationship and in 25% of cases, the parents had remarried and one parent was a stepparent to the children (see Table A.1). Ages of parents are found in Table A.2.

Seventy percent of the sample (31) was drawn from three different health centers. One center (Area 1) was located in a town in a rural area, a few hours drive from any major urban center. The other two centers were located in the metropolitan area of Sydney. Located in the outer western suburbs, Area 2 consisted of primarily low-income, blue-collar, and single-parent families, and was an area of high unemployment and a concentration of public housing. This area fell into the bottom one-fifth places in Sydney in terms of socioeconomic status. Area 3 was an established middle-distance suburb, consisting of both blue-collar and professional/managerial workers. Of the remaining 13 families, 3 were obtained from YACS, and 10 were obtained through other therapists from both high- and low-socioeconomic areas within Sydney metropolitan area. All but

TABLE A.1. Marital Status

	n	%
Married or *de facto*	15	34
Remarried	11	25
Separated/divorced	13	30
Never married or *de facto*	5	11
TOTALS	44	100

TABLE A.2. Age of Parent

	Mother	Father
Under 25	8	1
26–35	18	11
35–45	14	13
Over	45	4
TOTALS	44	27

three parents identified themselves as "Australian," that is, Australian-born of Australian parents (Horvath, 1986).

The research design had specifically included three different geographic areas representing a rural area, a lower-income suburb, and a middle-income suburb. It was in fact the case, however, that many of the families living in the middle-income areas were lower-income families, often living in public housing. Over half of the respondents relied on some sort of government social assistance, and less than half relied on employment income.

Those who were employed were from occupations typical of men and women in a working-class, gender-segregated labor market. Although only six women were engaged in paid work at the time of this study, and three had never been employed, most had worked at one time or another and had stopped work to care for their children. The majority had worked in low-paid, traditional female occupations including as cashiers, clerks, nursing aids, secretaries, receptionists, or waitresses. Seven stated they had worked in one of the following occupations: airline hostess, factory worker, kitchen worker, punch card operator, prostitute, seamstress, and teacher. All but six of the men had worked at some point in blue-collar or clerical occupations, including as clerk, bricklayer, butcher, cleaner, construction worker, gardener, laborer, mechanic, miner, panel beater, policeman, or truck driver. Five of these men were currently unemployed, and two described themselves as unemployable due to chronic illness or injury. Six men were engaged in professional or managerial occupations. Of these men, however, two fathers of adolescent daughters had not become clients of either therapists or YACS. Their daughters had left home following the disclosure of sexual assault and had sought therapy independently. Two other men were fathers of children who had been sexually assaulted by someone outside the family.

The great majority of parents had received less than 10 years of schooling, with only a small percentage reporting any education at the technical or university level (Table A.3).

In summary, more than one-third of the sample consisted of single-parent, woman-headed families. Over half the sample relied on social assistance, fewer than half were supported by the parents' employment, and fewer than one-third were supported by a parent employed in an occupation requiring any training or qualifications.

TABLE A.3. Parents' Educational Level

	Mother	Father
Under 10 years	27	20
10–12 years	11	1
Some technical or university	6	6
TOTALS	44	27

Types of Abuse

Therapists or D.O.s were asked in each case how they perceived the child to be at risk of abuse. In 43% of the cases referred to the study, one or both parents were allegedly abusive or at risk of abusing their child or children physically. In the four cases of more serious physical abuse involving fractures (in contrast to bruising), the father or stepfather was the alleged abuser. Twenty-seven percent of the parents (fathers or stepfathers) were allegedly abusive or at risk of abusing their children sexually. In approximately 14% of the cases, a child had disclosed sexual assault by someone outside of the family, and in 16%, a parent was perceived as not coping or as neglecting the children (see Table A.4).

Evidence of physical abuse included fractures, bruising, parents' disclosures that a child had been severely hit or beaten, or that an infant had been severely shaken. Sexual abuse was considered to be sexual contact between a child and person considerably older than the child. Sexual contact referred to activities engaged in for the sexual gratification of at least one person and ranged from nudity, exposure, and masturbation to oral–genital contact and anal and vaginal penetration.

Not coping or neglect referred to situations where the D.O. or therapist believed that parents were not providing adequate physical care or were at risk of physically abusing their children. Concern regarding the potential for physical abuse was most frequently generated by the mother's reports that she was "losing control" and feared assaulting her children or causing them physical harm.

Child sexual abuse differed from child physical abuse in several significant dimensions. First, physical abuse was more apparent and more easily "proven" than sexual abuse. Fractures, cuts, and bruises served as evidence. The majority of cases of sexual assault, on the other hand, provided no physical evidence and, in some cases, children's disclosures were denied by the perpetrators and disbelieved by others. Although physical abuse appeared to show no clear-cut gender preferences in terms of victims or perpetrators, sexual offenses, with two exceptions, were committed by men.

Last, allegations of physical abuse were less common in families within higher socioeconomic levels. Despite the fact that 43% of the cases concerned allegations of physical abuse, of the families with the highest education (some technical or university) and income levels, there was only one case of physical

TABLE A.4. Type of Abuse Allegations

Alleged abuse	Total	%
Physical	19	43
Sexual		
Intrafamilial	12	27
Interfamilial	6	14
Not coping or neglect	7	16
TOTALS	44	100

abuse. The rest represented cases of sexual assault, both interfamilial and intra-familial.

The families in this study had been involved with a number of agencies including YACS, health department therapists, other therapists, counselors from a school or preschool, hospital social workers, doctors, child health nurses, the police, and the courts. The number of agencies each family had been involved with ranged from 1 to 9, with an average of 4.45 and a median of 5. While this study focused primarily on family members' accounts of their experiences with D.O.s and therapists, for many, this represented only part of their experience with social and legal services.

METHOD OF ANALYSIS

The process of data analysis in this study corresponded most closely to the method described by Miles (1979), Glasser and Strauss (1967) and Glasser (1978). The process of analysis was ongoing and reflexive in the sense that analysis occurred after each interview and subsequently influenced what was sought and therefore analyzed in ensuing interviews. In this sense, data analysis proceeds, as Bulmer (1979, p. 653) put it, "Neither from observation to category, nor from category to observation, but in both directions at once and in interaction." Rather than testing a particular theory, the purpose of data analysis of this type is to generate theory that is grounded in the data.

The following suppositions, which were based on "hunches" from my clinical experience, influenced my early investigations. These were my beginning hypotheses:

1. Two factors that influence encounters between families and professionals are (a) whether parents feel coerced into involvement, and (b) whether or not professionals perceive the parents as compliant.

2. If families are notified to YACS and then ordered to therapy, therapists are more likely to perceive them as "resistant," and parents are likely to

perceive the D.O. (the frontline worker for YACS) and therapists negatively.

3. If parents refer themselves to YACS or to a therapist, they are more likely to be perceived as cooperative by professionals and to describe their relationship with professionals positively.

I undertook the analysis of research interviews in the following manner: Each research interview was transcribed shortly after the interview took place. In total, this resulted in approximately 1,440 double-spaced pages of text. Some time shortly after each interview, I read the interview text and, in some cases, listened again to the audiotape of the interview.

At this stage, I made notes on each transcript of recurring themes and key words used by participants (e.g., "Gestapo," "friend," "smacking," "bashing," "in control," "intrude," "judging," "taking sides," etc.). These are referred to as *first-order concepts*. As the number of interviews increased, I photocopied the transcripts and began to cut out the section of each transcript that referred to each of these first-order concepts. This ultimately resulted in a card box indexed according to the concept that gave me, for example, the section from every interview in which a participant had discussed the relationship with a professional in terms of "friend." This allowed me to compare the concept across cases.

I was at the same time monitoring the types of cases that the interviews represented and sought to increase the number of accounts in each of the four categories of "voluntary YACS," "involuntary YACS," "voluntary therapy," and "involuntary therapy."

	YACS	THERAPIST
VOLUNTARY		
INVOLUNTARY		

When there were a few cases in each of the aforementioned categories, I compared and contrasted the parents' accounts in each category. This was done on large sheets of paper, upon which I constructed grids representing each category, listed the families by name, and briefly encapsulated their accounts. This comparison and contrast ultimately yielded several propositions. These propositions, representing my conceptualization of the parents' accounts, I referred to as *second-order concepts*. Again, using grids on large sheets of paper, I tested these propositions by finding out in which cases the propositions held and in which they did not. When a proposition was found generally not to hold, it prompted further propositions. When it generally held, I looked in more detail at the exceptions to the rule. I then wrote notes summarizing the results indicating directions for future explorations (see Figure A.1).

Analysis: Ordered to Therapy
Proposition: Families that are ordered to therapy will undermine the referral by rejecting appointment times and not showing up for appointments.

1. Families ordered to therapy *did* attend when a child was removed, or when there was a threat to remove the children, *unless* the threat was not perceived as real, or unless the child had already been removed and the parents perceived little to gain from going to therapy in terms of having the child returned.

2. When parents were ordered, cooperation with the therapist was enhanced when parents perceived the therapist as on their side or the parents were offered some choice by the therapist.

3. Perhaps "Ordered to Therapy" or "Voluntary versus Involuntary" is not always so black and white. In some cases parents were not ordered (by the court or by threat from D.O.) but were referred, albeit reluctantly. Perhaps those situations in which the families do not show up or are inconsistent are really more "Reluctant Referrals," in that they were encouraged or urged rather than ordered to go to therapy.

4. Situations did not always remain clearly voluntary or involuntary, as in the case of the R. family, where the mother asked for help. The parents went to therapy voluntarily but were then ordered by YACS to attend (involuntarily).

FIGURE A.1. An example of a note concerning the question of "ordered to therapy."

Ultimately, many first-order concepts were processed similarly by comparing those situations in which the theme did or did not appear. Those situations that were shown to not fit the general rule prompted further rethinking of the material. When, for example, did parents ultimately trust therapists despite being ordered to therapy? When did parents see a D.O. as a friend, despite being notified to the Department?

Emerging concepts were further refined through three other means. First, because the interviews and the analysis proceeded simultaneously over a 2-year period, the understandings I developed at the earlier interviews were tested and clarified with parents in later interviews. This meant that over time, the interviews became progressively more able to confirm or reject the concepts I was developing. Second, once I had written draft chapters incorporating first-order concepts and clarified in my own mind many of my second-order concepts, I interviewed therapists and D.O.s, and contrasted their accounts with those of parents. Third, I gave draft chapters to several therapists and D.O.s to read and then discussed their responses with them.

I then returned to the transcripts of interviews with family members, and this time, rather than focusing on parents' descriptions of professionals, I looked for descriptions of their family and social contexts. Although this had not been the initial focus of my interviews, most participants had made reference to their situations through the course of the interview. In contrasting their accounts with the sociological research concerning working-class families, I was able to reconstruct a description of their contexts.

LIMITATIONS OF THIS STUDY

The findings of this study shed light on the context in which child abuse occurs and are significant for the theory and practice of family therapy and child abuse intervention. In contrast to what was originally envisioned, however, this research had several limitations. First, the sample was not a representative sample and was thus less inclusive than originally envisioned. Although I had sought to obtain "family members' " perceptions of intervention, the overwhelming majority of accounts were those from women. Most children were too young to be interviewed in depth, and some parents chose not to involve their children. In many cases, the women were single, separated, or divorced and living apart from their male partners. Even in those situations involving nuclear families, men were frequently not involved, or less involved, in therapy, and only the mother was interviewed.

Second, the sample was broader than simply "child-abusing" parents. Not all cases were confirmed cases of abuse—that is, registered by the Department following the investigation—and the sample also included families in which a child had been sexually abused by a neighbor or family friend. Although I was aware that such a broad definition might make it difficult to compare this study with others, the advantages of allowing a wider definition of abuse nevertheless appeared to outweigh the disadvantages. Child abuse is widely defined in practice, and "confirmation" and thus "registration" of abuse is often difficult. By allowing a broad definition of abuse, I have captured the experiences of many parents who were reported and investigated, despite the fact that their cases never reached "registration." I also obtained a cross section of cases seen by therapists in the public sector. Most important, by side-stepping the issues of who had abused and whether the abuse was confirmed or not, I avoided the vexed question of the truth of the allegations and the value judgments implied in any definition of abuse.

Last, the views of respondents in this study are likely to suffer from the problems of retrospective accounts. Given the nature of the allegations against some parents and the stigma inherent in the child abuse label, it is likely that their accounts are to some degree justifications or rationalizations of their own behavior after the fact. Nor could family members be aware of the extent to which therapists or child protection authority "personalities" were constrained by their own work context and policies. I do not mean to imply that there was an objective truth that could have been revealed but, rather, that the accounts given to me may to some extent have been reconstructions of the respondent's previous construction of the event. I would likely have received a different account had I had the opportunity to follow several cases over time, interviewing respondents after each of their encounters with District Officers and therapists. Although aware of these drawbacks, the clients' accounts, nevertheless, remained convincing to me, because they were backed up with details provided by others (e.g., a therapist's reports, a D.O.'s behavior, or vice versa), because of the repetition of themes across cases, and because their accounts corresponded to my observations as a therapist and supervisor.

References

Alderette, P., & deGraffenried, D. (1986) Nonorganic Failure-to-Thrive Syndrome and the Family System, *Child Abuse, 41*, 207–210.

Alexander, P. (1985) A Systems Theory Conceptualization of Incest, *Family Process, 24*, 79–88.

Almeida, R., Woods, R., Messineo, T., Font, R., & Heer, C. (1994) Violence in the Lives of the Racially and Sexually Different: A Public and Private Dilemma, *Journal of Feminist Family Therapy, 5*(3/4), 99–126.

Alpert, H. (Ed.) (1988) *We Are Everywhere: Writings by and about Lesbian Parents*, Crossing Press, Freedom, CA.

Amato, P. (1987) *Children in Australian Families: The Growth of Competence*, Prentice-Hall, Sydney.

Aponte, H. (1994) *Bread and Spirit: Therapy with the New Poor*, Norton, New York.

Aries, P. (1962) *Centuries of Childhood*, R. Baldick, trans., Jonathan Cape, London.

Bachrach, C. A. (1983) Children in Families: Characteristics of Biological, Step and Adopted Children, *Journal of Marriage and the Family, 45*, 171–179.

Berg, I. (1985) Helping Referral Sources Help, *Networker*, May–June, 59–65.

Bittman, M. (1991) *Juggling Time: How Australian Families Use Time*, Office of the Status of Women, Department of the Prime Minister and Cabinet, Canberra.

Boyd-Franklin, N. (1989) *Black Families in Therapy: A Multisystems Approach*, Guilford Press, New York.

Braverman, L. (1989) Beyond the Myth of Mothering, in M. McGoldrick, C. Anderson, & F. Walsh (Eds.), *Women in Families*, Norton: New York.

Bulmer, B. (1979) Concepts in the Analysis of Qualitative Data, *Sociological Review, 27*(4), 651–675.

Burns, A. (1986) Why Do Women Continue to Marry?, in M. Grieve & A.Burns (Eds.), *Australian Women: New Feminist Perspectives*, Oxford University Press, Oxford.

Carl, D., & Jurkovic, G. (1983) Agency Triangles: Problems in Agency–Family Relationships, *Family Process*, 22, 441–451.

Chodorow, N. (1978) *The Reproduction of Mothering: Psychoanalysis and the Sociology of Gender*, University of California Press, Berkley.

Cingolani, J. (1984) Social Conflict Perspective on Work with Involuntary Clients, *Social Work*, September–October, 442–446.

Clulow, C. (1993) New Families? Changes in Societies and Family Relationships, *Sexual and Marital Therapy*, 8(3), 269–273.

Cohen, T. (1983) The Incestuous Family Revisited, *Social Casework: The Journal of Contemporary Social Work*, 64, 154–161.

Connell, R. (1987) *Gender and Power*, Allen & Unwin, Sydney.

Corby, B. (1993) *Child Abuse: Towards a Knowledge Base*, Open University Press, Buckingham.

Coulton, C. J., Korbin, J. E., Su, M., & Chow, J. (1995) Community-Level Factors and Child Maltreatment Rates, *Child Development*, 66, 1262–1276.

Daly, M., & Wilson, M. I. (1994) Some Differential Attributes of Lethal Assaults on Small Children by Stepfathers versus Genetic Fathers, *Ethology and Sociobiology*, 15, 207–217.

Donaldson, N. (1991) *Time of Our Lives*, Allen & Unwin, Sydney.

Doughtery, N. (1983) The Holding Environment: Breaking the Cycle of Abuse, *Social Casework: The Journal of Contemporary Social Work*, 64, 283–288.

Dreyfus, H., & Rabinow, P. (1986) *Michel Foucault: Beyond Structuralism and Hermeneutics*, Harvester Press, Sussex, UK.

Dyche, L., & Zayas, L. (1995) The Value of Curiosity and Naivete for the Cross-Cultural Psychotherapist, *Family Process*, 34(4), 389–399.

Eckenrode, J., Levine-Powers, J., Doris, J., Munsch, J., & Bolger, N. (1986, August) *The Substantiation of Child Abuse and Neglect Reports*, paper presented at the Sixth International Conference on Child Abuse and Neglect, Sydney.

Edgar, D. (1980) *Introduction to Australian Society*, Prentice-Hall, Sydney.

Egeland, B. (1993) A History of Abuse is a Major Risk Factor for Abusing the Next Generation, in R. J. Gelles & D. R. Loseke (Eds.), *Current Controversies on Family Violence*, Sage, Newbury Park, CA.

Falicov, C. (1995) Training to Think Culturally: A Multidimentional Comparative Framework, *Family Process*, 34(4), 373–388.

Fine, M. (1993) Current Approaches to Understanding Family Diversity, *Family Relations*, 42, 235–237.

Foucault, M. (1980) Two Lectures, in *Power/Knowledge: Selected Interviews and Other Writings 1972–1977*, Pantheon Press, New York.

Foucault, M. (1984) Nietzsche, Genealogy, History, in P. Rabinow (Ed.), *The Foucault Reader*, Pantheon Press, New York.

Furniss, T. (1983) Mutual Influence and Interlocking Professional–Family Process in the Treatment of Child Sexual Abuse and Incest, *Child Abuse and Neglect*, 7, 207–223.

Gelles, R. J. (1973) Child Abuse as Psychopathology: A Sociological Critique and Reformulation, *American Journal of Orthopsychiatry*, 43(4), 611–621.

Gelles, R. J. (1975) The Social Construction of Child Abuse, *American Journal of Orthopsychiatry*, 45(3), 363–371.

Gelles, R. J. (1989) Child Abuse and Violence in Single-Parent Families: Parent Absence and Economic Deprivation, *American Journal of Orthopsychiatry*, 59(4), 492–501.

Gelles, R. J., & Straus, M. (1987) Is Violence towards Children Increasing? A Comparison of 1975 and 1985 National Survey Rates, *Journal of Interpersonal Violence*, 2(2), 212–222.

Gil, D. (1975) Unravelling Child Abuse, *American Journal of Orthopsychiatry*, 45(3), 346–356.

Gilding, M. (1991) *The Making and Breaking of the Australian Family*, Allen & Unwin, Sydney.

Glasser, B. G. (1978) *Theoretical Sensitivity: Advances in the Methodology of Grounded Theory*, Sociology Press, Mill Valley, CA.

Glasser, B. G., & Strauss, A. (1967) *The Discovery of Ground Theory: Strategies for Qualitative Research*, Deane, Chicago.

Goldner, V., Penn. P., Sheinberg, M., & Walker, G. (1990) Love and Violence: Gender Paradoxes in Volatile Attachments, *Family Process*, 29(4), 343–363.

Goode, W. (1982) Why Men Resist, in B. Thorne & M. Yalom (Eds.), *Rethinking the Family*, Longman, New York.

Graham, S. (1992) Most of the Subjects Were White and Middle-Class: Trends in Published Research on African-Americans in Selected A.P.A. Journals, 1970–1989, *American Psychologist*, 47, 629–639.

Grosz, E. (1989) *Sexual Subversions*, Allen & Unwin, Sydney.

Gutheil, T., & Avery, N. (1977) Multiple Overt Incest as Family Defense against Loss, *Family Process*, 16(1), 105–116.

Hall, R., & Greene, B. (1994) Cultural Competence in Feminist Family Therapy: An Ethical Mandate, *Journal of Feminist Family Therapy*, 6(3), 5–28.

Hardy, K., & Laszloffy, T. (1994) Deconstructing Race in Family Therapy, *Journal of Feminist Family Therapy*, 5(3/4), 5–33.

Hare-Mustin, R. (1994) Sex, Lies and Headaches: The Problem Is Power, in T. Goodrich (Ed.), *Women's Power*, Norton, New York.

Henggeler, S., & Borduin, C. (1990) *Family Therapy and Beyond: A Multisystemic Approach to Treating Behavior Problems of Children and Adolescents*, Brooks/Cole, Pacific Grove, CA.

Ho, C. (1990) An Analysis of Domestic Violence in Asian American Communities: A Multicultural Approach to Counselling, in L. Brown & P. Root (Eds.), *Diversity and Complexity in Feminist Therapy*, Haworth Press, New York.

Horvath, R. (1986) Socio-Spacial Inequality in Australia, in J. B. McLoughlin & M. Huxley (Eds.), *Urban Planning in Australia: Critical Readings*, Longman Cheshire, Melbourne.

Imber-Black, E. (1988) *Families and Larger Systems: A Family Therapist's Guide through the Labyrinth*, Guilford Press, New York.

James, K., & McIntyre, D. (1982) The Reproduction of Families: The Social Role of Family Therapy, *Journal of Marriage and Family Therapy*, 9, 19–129.

James, K., & MacKinnon, L. (1990) The "Incestuous Family" Revisited: A Critical Analysis of Family Therapy Myths, *Journal of Marital and Family Therapy, 16*(1), 71–88.

Jayaratne, S. (1977) Child Abusers as Parents and Children: A Review, *Social Work,* January, 5–9.

Katz, M., Hampton, R., Newberger, E., Bowles, R., & Snyder, J. (1986) Returning Children Home: Clinical Decision Making in Cases of Child Abuse and Neglect, *American Journal of Orthopsychiatry, 56*(2), 253–262.

Kaufman, J., & Ziegler, E. (1987) Do Abused Children Become Abusive Parents? *American Journal of Orthopsychiatry, 57*(2), 186–192.

Kempe, R., & Kempe, C. (1978) *Child Abuse,* Harvard University Press, Cambridge, MA.

Kitzinger, C. (1987) *The Social Construction of Lesbianism,* Sage, London.

Kleinberg, S. (1979) Success and the Working Class, *Journal of American Culture, 2*(1), 123–138.

Langeland, W., & Dijkstra, F. (1995) Breaking the Intergenerational Transmission of Child Abuse: Beyond the Mother–Child Relationship, *Child Abuse Review, 4*(1), 4–13.

Lau, A. (1986) Family Therapy across Cultures, in J. L. Cox (Ed.), *Transcultural Psychiatry,* Croom Helm, London.

Lee, E. (1990) Family Therapy with Southeast Asian Families, in M. Mirkin (Ed.), *The Social and Political Contexts of Family Therapy,* Allyn & Bacon, Needham Heights, MA.

Luepnitz, D. (1988) *The Family Interpreted,* Basic Books, New York.

MacKinnon, L. (1992) *Child Abuse in Context: The Participants' View,* PhD dissertation, University of Sydney.

MacKinnon, L. (1993) Systems in Settings: Therapist as Power Broker, *Australian and New Zealand Journal of Family Therapy, 14*(3), 117–122.

Magura, S., & Moses, B. (1984) Clients as Evaluators in Child Protective Services, *Child Welfare, 63*(2), 99–112.

Malick, M., & Ardi, A. (1981) Politics of Interprofessional Collaboration: Challenge to Advocacy, *Social Casework, 62,* 122–127.

Martin, H. (1984) Intervention with Infants at Risk for Abuse or Neglect, *Child Abuse and Neglect, 8,* 255–260.

Matthews, J. (1984) *Good and Mad Women: The Historical Construction of Femininity in 20th Century Australia,* Allen & Unwin, Sydney.

McGill, D. (1992) The Cultural Story in Multicultural Family Therapy: Families in Society, *Journal of Contemporary Human Services,* June, 339–349.

McGoldrick, M. (1994) Family Therapy: Having a Place Called Home, *Journal of Feminist Family Therapy, 5*(3/4), 127–156.

McNeil, J., & McBride, M. (1979) Group Therapy with Abusive Parents, *Social Casework: The Journal of Contemporary Social Work, 60,* 36–42.

McRobbie, A. (1978) Working-Class Girls and the Culture of Femininity, in Women's Study Group (Eds.), *Women Take Issue: Aspects of Women's Subordination,* University of Birmingham Press, London.

Miles, M. (1979) Qualitative Data as an Attractive Nuisance: The Problem of Analysis, *Administrative Science Quarterly, 24,* 590–601.

Milner, J. S., & Chilamkurti, C. (1991) Physical Child Abuse Perpetrator Characteristics: A Review of the Literature, *Journal of Interpersonal Violence*, 6, 345–366.

National Research Council (1993) *Understanding Child Abuse and Neglect*, National Academy Press, Washington, DC.

Newberger, E. (1983) The Helping Hand Strikes Again: Unintended Consequences of Child Abuse Reporting, *Journal of Clinical Child Psychology*, 12(3), 307–310.

Parton, N. (1985) *The Politics of Child Abuse*, Macmillan, London.

Pelton, L. (1978) Child Abuse and Neglect: The Myth of Classlessness, *American Journal of Orthopsychiatry*, 48(4), 608–617.

Pinderhughes, E. (1989) *Understanding Race, Ethnicity and Power*, Simon & Schuster, New York.

Pinderhughes, E. (1990) Legacy of Slavery: The Experience of Black Families in America, in M. Mirkin (Ed.), *The Social and Political Contexts of Family Therapy*, Allyn & Bacon, Needham Heights, MA.

Ransom, D. (1982) Resistance: Family- or Therapist-Generated?, in A. Gurman (Ed.), *Questions and Answers in the Practice of Family Therapy*, Vol. II, Brunner/Mazel, New York.

Rubin, L. B. (1992) *Worlds of Pain: Life in the Working-Class Family*, Basic Books, New York.

Rich, A. (1980) Compulsory Heterosexuality and Lesbian Existence, *Signs: Journal of Women in Culture and Society*, 5(4), 631–60.

Sack, W., Mason, R., & Higgins, J. (1985) The Single Parent Family and Abusive Child Punishment, *American Journal of Orthopsychiatry*, 55(2), 253–259.

Salter, A., Richardson, C., & Martin, P. (1985) Treating Abusive Parents, *Child Welfare*, 64(4), 327–341.

Samuel, L. (1983) The Making of a School Resister: A Case Study of Australian Working Class Secondary School Girls, in R. Browne & L. Foster (Eds.), *Sociology of Education*, 3rd ed., Macmillan, Melbourne.

Scutt, J. (1983) *Even in the Best of Homes*, Penguin Books, Ringwood, Victoria.

Sennett, R., & Cobb, J. (1972) *The Hidden Injuries of Class*, Cambridge University Press, London.

Sgroi, S. (1982) *Handbook of Clinical Intervention in Child Sexual Abuse*, Lexington Books, Lexington, MA.

Sheinberg, M. (1992) Navigating Treatment Impasses at the Disclosure of Incest: Combining Ideas from Feminism and Social Constructionism, *Family Process*, 31(3), 201–216.

Sheinberg, M., True, F., & Fraenkel, P. (1994) Treating the Sexually Abused Child: A Recursive Multimodal Program, *Family Process*, 33(3), 263–276.

Smith, S. (1984), Significant Research Findings in The Etiology of Child Abuse, *Social Casework: The Journal of Contemporary Social Work*, 65(6), 337–346.

Spinetta, J., & Rigler, D. (1972) The Child Abusing Parent: A Psychological Review, *Psychological Bulletin*, 77(4), 296–304.

Spurkland, I., & Koppang, B. (1985) Family Admittance for Assessment of Child Abuse/Neglect, Problems in Co-operation between Local Agencies and the Family Wards, *Acta Paedopsychiatrica*, 6, 67–73.

Star, B. (1980) Patterns in Family Violence, *Social Casework: The Journal of Contemporary Social Work, 61,* 339–346.

Strube, M., & Barbour, L. (1983) The Decision to Leave an Abusive Relationship: Economic Dependence and Psychological Commitment, *Journal of Marriage and the Family,* November, 785–793.

Susman, E., Trickett, P., Iannotti, R., Hollenbeck, G., & Zahn-Waxler, C. (1985) Child-Rearing Patterns in Depressed, Abusive, and Normal Mothers, *American Journal of Orthopsychiatry, 55*(2), 237–251.

Taylor, R. (1984) Marital Therapy in the Treatment of Incest, *Social Casework: The Journal of Contemporary Social Work, 65,* 195–202.

Tuszynski, A. (1985) Group Treatment That Helps Abusive or Neglectful Parents, *Social Casework: The Journal of Contemporary Social Work, 66,* 556–562.

van Krieken, R. (1986) Beyond Social Control, *Theory and Society, 15,* 401–429.

Viaro, M., & Peruzzi, P. (1983) Home Visits in Crisis Situations: Analysis of Context and Suggestions for Intervention, *Australian Journal of Family Therapy,* 4(4), 209–215.

Vinson, T. (1987, April 15) *Child Abuse and the Media,* paper presented at Sydney University of Criminology Seminar.

Wearing, B. (1984) *The Ideology of Motherhood,* Allen & Unwin, Sydney.

Webster-Stratton, C. (1985) Comparison of Abusive and Nonabusive Families with Conduct-Disordered Children, *American Journal of Orthopsychiatry, 55*(1), 59–69.

Western, J. (1983) *Social Inequality in Australian Society,* Macmillan, Melbourne.

Weston, K. (1991) *Families We Choose: Lesbians, Gays, Kinship,* Columbia University Press, New York.

Wilkinson, M. (1987) *An Examination of Practice in Substitute Care in the 1960's,* unpublished master's thesis, Department of Social Work and Social Policy, University of Sydney.

Wolfe, D. (1984) Treatment of Abusive Parents: A Reply to the Special Issue, *Journal of Clinical Child Psychology, 13*(2), 192–194.

Wolock, I., & Horowitz, B. (1984) Child Maltreatment as a Social Problem: The Neglect of Neglect, *American Journal of Orthopsychiatry, 54*(4), 530–543.

Wooley, P., & Evans, W. (1955) Significance of Skeletal Lesions in Infants Resembling Those with Traumatic Origin, *Journal of the American Medical Association, 174,* 158–165.

Zuelzer, M., & Reposa, R. (1983) Mothers in Incestuous Families, *International Journal of Family Therapy, 5*(2), 98–109.

Index

The abbreviation (fn) following a page number indicates footnote material.
(T) refers to tables and (F) to figures.

DATE